COMPARATIVE GUIDE
TO
CHILDREN'S
NUTRITIONALS

A Compendium of Products Available in the United States and Canada

by

Lyle MacWilliam, BSc, MSc, FP

Second Edition

Copy Editing
Arlene MacWilliam

Research, Editing and Layout
Gregg Gies

Cover Design
Ian Black, MGDC

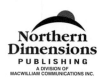

Northern Dimensions
PUBLISHING
A DIVISION OF
MACWILLIAM COMMUNICATIONS INC.

Comparative Guide to Children's Nutritionals
A Compendium of Products Available in the United States and Canada

Published by Northern Dimensions Publishing
a division of MacWilliam Communications Inc.
Vernon, British Columbia, CANADA
www.northerndimensions.com

This comparative guide is produced for educational and comparative purposes only. No person should use the information herein for self-diagnosis, treatment or justification in accepting or declining any medical treatment for any health-related problems. Some medical therapies, including the use of medicines, may be affected by the use of certain nutritional supplements. Therefore, any individual with a specific health problem should seek advice by a qualified medical practitioner before starting a supplementation program. The decision whether to consume any nutritional supplement rests with the individual, in consultation with his or her medical advisor. Furthermore, nothing in this manual should be misinterpreted as medical advice.

This comparative guide is intended to assist in sorting through the maze of nutritional supplements available in the marketplace today. It is not a product endorsement and does not make any health claim, other than to document recent findings in the scientific literature. This comparative guide was not commissioned by any public sector or private sector interest, or by any company whose products may be represented in this document. The research, development and findings are the sole creative effort of MacWilliam Communications Inc.

Neither the publisher nor the author may be held responsible for the accuracy of information provided by or obtained from third parties, including but not limited to information gathered from nutritional supplement companies, medical and scientific journals, newspapers, magazines and/or Internet web sites.

Library and Archives Canada Cataloguing in Publication

MacWilliam, Lyle Dean
      Comparative guide to children's nutritionals : a compendium of products
available in the United States and Canada / by Lyle MacWilliam ; copy editing, Arlene MacWilliam ; research, editing and layout, Gregg Gies ; cover design, Ian Black.

Includes bibliographical references.
ISBN 0-9732538-1-9

      1. Dietary supplements. 2. Children--Nutrition. I. MacWilliam, Arlene
II. Gies, Gregg III. Title.

RJ53.V57M32 2004   615'.328'083   C2004-905323-X

Dedication

To my children, Laurie, Matthew, Tana and Karalyn

Before I had children, I had four terrific theories about parenting.
Now, I have four terrific children—and no theories.

With Thanks

This book is the culmination of years of effort in developing the scientific rationale, and in refining and enhancing the analytical models used to conduct our comparative analysis. With each edition, we have built on our previous work in order to provide consumers with a comprehensive, up-to-date and reliable source of information on the science of nutritional supplementation and the products available. In doing so, we have, admittedly, stood on the shoulders of others; the insights, knowledge and guidance gleaned from the scientific authorities we have referenced in developing our analytical models have been invaluable resources.

I am deeply indebted to my wife, Arlene, who has patiently endured my emotional highs and lows as I have struggled to pull together a seemingly endless volume of scientific and product research. Her sharp editorial eye, unwavering demand for rigor, and her innate ability to bring me back to center have ensured the quality of this creative effort.

I am also indebted to my associate, Gregg Gies, a true master in the science of Information Technology and a tireless researcher whose ability to ferret out information knows no bounds. As the technical and creative director, Gregg's hand is written large throughout this publication.

To Ian Black of Ian Black Concepts, I owe a heartfelt "thank you." Ian's extensive talents in developing the cover design and the creative aspects of the publication have provided immeasurable value to the finished work.

Last, but certainly not least, my thanks to you, the purchaser of this guide, for your support. In particular, I am grateful to those of my readership who have provided feedback on previous editions of this guide; the encouragement, support and constructive criticism received from so many of you continue to inspire me to reach beyond myself, in what has truly become a labor of love. Thank you.

May health be your constant companion.

Lyle

September, 2004

TABLE OF CONTENTS

I saw few die of hunger; of eating, a hundred thousand.
—*Benjamin Franklin (1706 - 1790)*

CHAPTER ONE

INVESTING IN THEIR FUTURE

Nutrition plays a key role in everyone's health, especially that of our children. Because of the nutrient demands of their rapidly developing bodies, it is essential that young people receive adequate amounts of the nutrients they require for optimal growth and development.

However, our children seem to be growing "largely" in the wrong direction: obesity has become the most common nutritional disease among children and adolescents in both Canada and the United States.[1] Consequently, those degenerative diseases related to overweight and obesity are plaguing people of all ages, striking sooner in life than ever before. As in adults, simply being overweight or obese can significantly elevate the risk of degenerative disease in a young person.[2] In fact, excess abdominal weight is a key risk factor for the development of cardiovascular disease and diabetes in later life.[3,4]

A virtual revolution in both eating habits and physical activity is essential to restore health to our youth. Because of the conveniences of our modern world, many children are now consuming a diet that is more harmful than healthful. As a society, we are raising our children on calorie-laden junk food: food high in salt, hydrogenated fats and sugars; food stripped of much of its nutritional value through over-processing; food laced with pesticides, preservatives and artificial colourings. Our children have also become soft: their ballooning waistlines are testimony to their chronic "couch-potatoism." While naturally more active than adults, today's kids the world over are spending far too much of their free time watching television and playing video games—time that ought to be spent building strong bones. The consequences are flabby bellies, soggy butts and cardiovascular systems that are prematurely showing signs of serious damage.

Overfed and Undernourished

It wasn't always this way. Despite the years of post-war austerity, young children of the forties and fifties ate a much healthier diet when compared to kids of the nineties. In a recent longitudinal study, Prynne and co-workers[5] compared the diets of children in the 1990s to those of children in the 1950s. Their findings reveal that the diet of an average four-year-old in 1950 contained more breads, grains and vegetables and far less refined sugar. Raw fibre and calcium intakes were markedly higher and tea was the most common drink. Today, soft drinks, scarce in the fifties, are consumed by 90 percent of today's kids. Back in the 1950s most of the vitamin C came from natural sources; today's kids regularly get their C with their soft-drink sugar "fix." Refined sugar has replaced starch as *the* major energy source for growing bodies.

On this the science is clear: the dietary and lifestyle choices of today's children are placing them on a fast track to degenerative

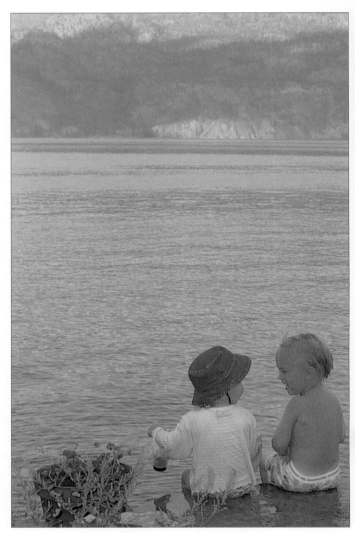

disease.[6] Diabetes, cardiovascular disease, pulmonary disorders, osteoarthritis, osteoporosis, non-alcoholic fatty liver disease[7] and cancer threaten to rob them of their quality of life down the road.

Research also shows that a proper nutritional foundation at an early age can be a resilient buttress for lifelong health; unfortunately, the reverse is also true. The fact is, active participation in sports is giving way to the sedentary nature of computers and gaming systems; candies and sweets are replacing fruits and vegetables as snacks; and soda pop has replaced milk, juices and water as the youngsters' beverage of choice. Health and longevity are being traded off for convenience and comfort—and the consequences are stark.

The irony is that today we have access to a far greater variety of fresh produce than most families had in the middle of the 20th century. Unfortunately, our access to heavily refined foods and empty calories is even greater. As parents, we need to change this balance through consumer demand: choose mainly fresh, organic fruits and vegetables, whole grains, legumes and dairy products. Reject processed foods, particularly those laden with fats and sugars. Please, don't compromise the health of your children. Teach them the importance of a healthful diet and the value of regular exercise—then practise what you teach.

Patterns in Infancy

According to the International Food Information Council,[8] the patterns of diet and exercise that develop during childhood cast the mold for lifelong habits that can lead to health or infirmity in later years. These patterns have a strong correlation with later cognitive development[9,10] and the protection against degenerative disease. For example, it is generally accepted that breastfeeding has many benefits for infants, in particular the reduction of cholesterol levels and other cardiovascular disease risk factors that become manifest later in life.[11] There are also indications that breastfeeding children longer than twelve months may significantly reduce their future risk of obesity[12] and type 2 diabetes.[13]

> *Research shows that a proper nutritional foundation at an early age can be a resilient buttress for lifelong health; unfortunately, the reverse is also true.*

Further evidence that sound nutrition and fitness habits can last a lifetime is provided in a recent study on nutritional programming.[14] The findings reveal that children, during their early development, have sensitive windows for nutritional programming. Dietary patterns established during these critical periods appear to imprint long-term consequences. This is confirmed in a recent study, which showed that obesity is directly related to birth weight and childhood growth rates.[15] Another study, of North American Indian five-year-olds, found that early obesity was the dominant risk factor for obesity later in youth.[16]

In Finland, relationships were found between the subsequent development of type 2 diabetes and fetal growth rates, rapid weight gain in infancy, and *late adiposity rebound* (the later recovery of "baby fat" after its initial diminishing around age two).[17] More disconcerting are recent findings showing that obese adolescents are more likely to develop degenerative diseases as adults *even* if they later lose the excess weight.[18] Unquestionably, being a chubby chick in your youth can spell big trouble down the road.

Nutritional Markers

Birth weight and weight at one year, now regarded as key nutritional indicators, are predictive markers for cardiovascular disease[19] and type 2 diabetes[20] in adulthood. The findings are supported by epidemiological data (information gathered from large populations) that link early nutritional habits to the later onset of cardiovascular disease and related risk factors. Families with a history of cardiovascular disease should also keep an eye on the weight of their children, as some studies indicate that children in these families are more likely to have a high body mass index and become obese, hypertensive and diabetic.[21]

These risks do not develop independently of one another. An overweight or obese child increases his or her risk of developing a multitude of related ailments. Autopsies conducted as part of the Bogalusa Heart Study provide evidence that atherosclerotic plaques in coronary arteries increase dramatically along with the presence of other markers of metabolic syndrome (the precursor to frank diabetes), such as hyperinsulinemia (high blood insulin levels), hypertension (high blood pressure) and central-body obesity.[22]

Curiously, parents of children with low birth weights must also be vigilant.[23] Levitt and Lambert[24] found compelling evidence, based on epidemiological studies, that unusually small size at birth in full-term pregnancies is linked with the subsequent development of the major features of metabolic syndrome, namely glucose intolerance, hyperinsulinemia, hyptertension, disturbances in lipid metabolism, and increased mortality from cardiovascular disease.

The fetus appears to respond to metabolic insults during the prenatal growth period through the process of "programming." While this confers short-term survival advantages, there may be a long-term disadvantage in that it is associated with cardiovascular disease, hypertension, type 2 diabetes, and later obesity. What's more, such programming can impact the aging process itself. A possible causal mechanism linking early growth variations to later chronic disease risk through telomeric* attrition has been identified. The shortening of telomeric DNA with each cell division serves as a type of biological clock and marks the rate of growth and repair within the cell. It is believed that telomeric alterations due to fetal growth variations may impact cellular senescence (aging) and affect not only lifelong cellular division, but also relative growth rates and degenerative disease processes.[25]

Setting an Example

Many parents who take their children out for dinner at the local fast-food watering hole are not likely to consider that the day-to-day nutritional choices they make for their children—even before birth—will later affect their health as an adult.[26] The evidence clearly shows that nutritional and fitness habits established during childhood *will* last a lifetime.

For any caring parent, these findings present an onerous responsibility that starts right from conception. How you feed your children today will determine their susceptibility to degenerative disease tomorrow—ample reason that the focus of childhood nutrition *must* be to promote optimal growth and development by building sound dietary patterns right from the get-go.[27]

The next time you are temped to settle for a fast-food fix for the kids at your local "greasy spoon," remember this: fast foods are a false economy. They may be a convenience now, but they come at a steep price to your children's health later.

---

* At the ends of each of our 23 pairs of chromosomes are tiny molecular "caps" called telomeres, which act much like the protective caps on the ends of our shoelaces. Telomeres play an important role in cell division and longevity. Each time a cell replicates, the telomere caps shorten until, after approximately 50 divisions, they reach a critical length. This signals a period of cellular senescence followed by death. Many scientists believe telomeres to be the biological clock which controls aging.

The Obesity Connection

Adolescent obesity is among the most pressing of medical problems in North America today. In a study reported in the *Archives of Pediatrics and Adolescent Medicine*, it was found that 22 percent of the 2300 children and adolescents surveyed fit the criteria for overweight—up 15 percent from a survey taken only three years earlier.[28]

In developed countries, the problem appears more prevalent among lower income groups. Worldwide prevalence for obesity ranges from a low of 2.6 percent in Finland, to 16 percent in Singapore. In the United States, it was found to be 11 percent.[29]

As if to further complicate matters, a recent study on weight concerns and smoking initiation revealed that, among both girls and boys, the contemplation of smoking and experimentation with cigarettes is positively related to weight-control behaviors and unhappiness with body image.[30]

As disconcerting as these facts may be, what is even more worrisome is the recent finding that the prenatal period and early adolescence appear to demarcate critical imprinting periods for the entrainment of obesity into adulthood.[31] There may even be neural circuits in the brain, at least in those genetically predisposed to obesity, that become "hardwired" to accept overweight or obesity as the norm when excess weight is maintained over time.[32] This metabolic imprinting makes it even more difficult to maintain a lower body weight because the brain defends against weight loss below a threshold that it has learned to accept as normal.

Few studies have examined the long-term consequences of childhood obesity on adult disease; however, childhood obesity does appear to increase the probability of adult morbidity and mortality. In a 1998 study by Dietz,[33] it was found that morbidity and mortality from colon cancer and cardiovascular disease were elevated in men who were obese during adolescence. Among both men and women with a history of obesity, rates of cardiovascular disease and diabetes were significantly increased. Several other studies confirm that avoiding childhood obesity may be the best insurance to prevent future hypertension and hyperlipidemia (high blood fats). Encouraging healthy eating patterns and daily physical activities are considered essential.[34,35,36]

Obesity is consistently linked to the development of several degenerative diseases in adults. Caballero found that, while preventive intervention to curb obesity in adult life may reduce risk, it is usually difficult and results are often limited. In contrast, interventions early in life could result in major reductions in the incidence of several diseases in adulthood.[37] Some researchers speculate that obesity acts as an inflammatory condition, raising the blood levels of inflammatory markers such as C-reactive protein, which is associated with cardiovascular disease and other degenerative processes.[38]

Worldwide, both childhood and adult obesity are increasing at alarming rates, but childhood obesity has the potential to be far more devastating since it puts risk factors in place at the same time that young bodies are growing and changing. In addition to North America,[39] regions with diverse food sources and lifestyles, including Australia,[40] Egypt,[41] Mexico,[42] Europe[43,44,45] and Asia,[46,47,48] all report marked increases in degenerative disease—particularly type 2 diabetes and cardiovascular disease—coupled with rapid rises in obesity rates. Many researchers believe that the shift away from traditional diets to a high-fat, sugar-laden "western" diet is the major reason for these changes.[49] In Baja California, Mexican children now consume very low quantities of fruits and vegetables and excessive amounts of high-fat snacks and soft drinks.[50] Ninety-two percent of fifth graders consume at least one soft drink daily, and most (85 percent) also consume at least one high-fat snack. This potentially deadly combination of high-sugar and high-fat intake is putting children directly in harm's way.

Other trends often associated with western culture are showing up around the world. In Iranian adolescents, a 2003 study revealed rapidly growing levels of obesity; the levels were associated with increased intakes of high-carbohydrate foods like white rice, pasta, bread, fast foods and foods high in salt.[51] Researchers also found that obese Iranian youths watch more television and participate in fewer sporting activities than their thinner peers. Other trends correlate with findings elsewhere in the world: girls tend to be more obese and more likely to develop type 2 diabetes than boys.[52,53,54,55,56] Researchers often suggest cultural factors, particularly sports participation, as possible contributors to the gender differences in the development of overweight, obesity and type 2 diabetes. Urban youth are more obese than rural youth,[57] and wealthy, well-educated parents are less likely to raise obese children than poor or uneducated parents, particularly single mothers.[58]

In some cases, premature adrenarche (sometimes called early puberty and primarily marked by the development of pubic hair, armpit hair or body odor prior to the age of eight years) may be the result of metabolic syndrome. A study of African-American and Hispanic girls found that premature adrenarche was most common in obese girls with higher degrees of hyperinsulinism and insulin resistance,[59] which can in turn lead to hyperandrogenism (development of male-like sexual characteristics). Many of these girls also had a family history of type 2 diabetes.

There appear to be ethnic patterns as well, with African-American, Hispanic and Native American children often showing higher rates of obesity and type 2 diabetes than other American children.[60,61,62,63] Again, girls appear to be affected more often than boys, particularly during adolescence.[64]

A Societal Problem

Researchers note that our obesity epidemic is a societal problem, not just an individual affliction. To keep our children healthy, families as a whole need to be better educated in healthy

> *Metabolic imprinting makes it even more difficult to maintain a lower body weight because the brain defends against weight loss below a threshold that it has learned to accept as normal.*

> *To keep our children healthy, families need to be better educated in healthy lifestyle choices, including food choices, meal preparation, exercise requirements and the myriad dangers of becoming overweight.*

**Ask your child what he wants for dinner
only if he's buying.**

—Fran Lebowitz (1950 -)

<u>CHAPTER TWO</u>

THE NEED FOR SUPPLEMENTATION

Nothing can replace the value of regular exercise and an active lifestyle, complemented with sound nutrition through a carefully balanced diet. This is the way Nature intended it to be. Unfortunately, children (and adults) in today's high-stress world face a dearth of beneficial physical activity and a steady diet of meals on the run—fast-food restaurants and processed foods, devoid of nutritional value. It is the exception, rather than the rule, that kids today will sit down to home-cooked meals with fresh-from-the-garden fruits and vegetables served up with loving care. Even for those fortunate enough to do so, there is no guarantee that they are receiving all the nutrients they need.

Children's Nutrition Today

While kids are beginning to understand the basic tenets of healthy eating—variety, balance and moderation—they don't make the grade when it comes to understanding what constitutes "good nutrition." A U.S. Department of Agriculture report to Congress noted only two percent of children and adolescents meet the nutritional recommendations for the five food groups (fruit, grains, meat, dairy and vegetables);[1] however, most consume 20 percent of their calories from the "Fats, Oils and Sweets" tip of the food guide pyramid, contributing to a deficiency of many nutrients, including iron, vitamin A, vitamin B$_6$ and calcium.[2]

This same pattern of high-fat, high-sugar consumption is noted in the USDA Continuing Survey of Food Intakes (1998).[3] The survey reveals the following:

✔ consumption of fruit declines with age;

✔ while 75 percent of all children eat at least one vegetable on a given day, their favourite is potatoes—french-fried or as processed potato chips;

✔ fewer than 16 percent eat corn or legumes on a given day and this percentage drops even lower for dark green or yellow vegetables;

✔ consumption of non-citrus juice mixes is up 280 percent from the previous survey;

✔ children and teens are socking back soft drinks—intake tripled since 1978, with nearly 75 percent of teenage boys consuming an average of three cans of soda each day;

✔ among children five or under, the consumption of soft drinks rose 16 percent and milk consumption plummeted dramatically across all age groups;

✔ by their teens, fast-food restaurants are the most frequent venue for adolescents when eating away from home; and,

✔ while children and teenage boys meet their daily nutritional requirements for most nutrients, teenage girls meet less than

86% of the daily requirements for calcium, magnesium, zinc and vitamin E.

Setting a Poor Example

Our public school systems play a vital role in molding children's attitudes and behaviors about nutrition and physical activity. In fact, a 1994 Gallup Poll conducted in the United States revealed that schools and teachers were considered the primary sources of nutritional information for 90 percent of the students surveyed.

Unfortunately, our schools have not helped our children make healthier choices. While some physical education and life skills courses have focussed on nutrition and exercise, administrative choices have undermined these efforts. To help shore up funding shortfalls, most schools have installed vending machines that tempt kids with high-sugar chocolate bars, fat-laden potato chips, sodium-laced pretzels and other treats that provide little nutritional value and contribute to the development of metabolic syndrome, the precursor of type 2 diabetes.

Washington, DC's Center for Science in the Public Interest (CSPI) recently published a report condemning schools that line their hallways—and their pockets—with vending machines selling junk food and soda pop to students.[4] Their survey of schools across America revealed that most choices presented in school vending machines are poor nutritional choices. In middle and high schools, for example, 80 percent of vending machine slots stocked candy, potato chips or sweet baked goods. More telling, and devastating to the health of our children, *less than half of one percent* of slots offered a fruit or vegetable. The findings for beverage choices were similar: almost three-quarters of all vending machine slots featured sugar-filled drinks like soda pop, sweetened or artificial fruit drinks and iced tea. Less than seven percent were real, unsweetened fruit choices and only five percent of offerings were milk—less than half of those dairy choices were skim or low-fat milk. CSPI notes in its report that the U.S. Department of Agriculture recommends nutritious choices for school meal programs, though it does not have the authority to enforce those recommendations.

So, what message do we send our youth when schools hallways are cluttered with pop machines and junk food dispensers? What is our nutritional message to them when, as parents, we march them off to a fast-food restaurant for the "real meal deal." We're letting our young people down – and they'll be the ones to pay the price.

Fortunately, some schools are beginning to take obesity and the problem of junk food seriously. In Texas, sales of all junk foods are prohibited on school property during lunch hours[5] and, since 2002, some of the largest school districts in the United States have banned soda pop from vending machines, replacing these high-sugar beverages with juices and bottled water. Los Angeles, Chicago and New York boards are among the leaders in this effort, and are following up with junk-food vending bans beginning in 2004.

Some school boards are resisting this change to healthier foods and beverages in vending machines. They fear students will purchase fewer products, leading to an increase in funding shortfalls. However, CSPI reports that the opposite appears to be the case: schools moving to healthier choices noticed little drop in revenues and, in at least one case (Venice High School in Los Angeles), revenues from snack sales *doubled* in the student store in the two years following the change.[6]

Depleted Soils, Depleted Foods

Today, relatively few families in Canada and America can boast garden-fresh produce. Most shoppers must rely on commercial agriculture to meet their daily nutritional needs. Yet, for the last 50 years, most commercial farms have relied on chemical fertilizers to grow their crops. During the late forties, three minerals, nitrogen (N), phosphorus (P) and potassium (K), (left over from the World War II armaments industry) were found to produce fine looking crops. The subsequent use of these nutrients quickly replaced traditional mulching and manuring. Decades of misuse has depleted North American soils of many of the essential micronutrients.[7]

To make things worse, commercial processing of these already nutrient-deficient foods further depletes their nutritional value. The mass production processes of storing, drying, cooking, freeze-drying, extracting and hydrogenating wreak havoc on an already marginal nutrient content. According to Dr. Michael Colgan, the processing of cereal grains depletes the magnesium content by 80 percent. Up to 50 percent of the folic acid content in foods is lost through preparation, processing and storage, while commercial milling of cereals depletes the vitamin B_6 content by 50 to 90 percent. Store asparagus for a week and 90 percent of its vitamin C is gone; blanch vegetables or fish and up to one-half of their B-complex vitamins and vitamin C content is lost.[8, 9,10]

Even with the best of intentions and the most careful planning, daily consumption of commercially processed foods grown in nutrient-deficient soils will not provide us with the quality nutrition we need for a lifetime of optimal health. The simple fact of the matter is, if the nutrients are not in the soil and not in our foods, then they're *not* in our bodies.

It Pays to Take Your Vitamins

While few of us have the time—or the available space—to grow our own natural food sources, there is a simple and effective means of ensuring that your children's daily nutritional needs are met. In addition to providing them with the most nutritious meals possible, give them a high quality, broad-spectrum nutritional supplement containing a *balanced* blend of the required vitamins, minerals and antioxidants necessary for optimal health. Supplementation adds back to our diets many of the micronutrients now lacking in our food supply. These nutrients serve as essential components in the metabolic processes that maintain the health of our cells.

After 20 years, the American Medical Association (AMA) has completely reversed its anti-vitamin stance and now encourages all adults to supplement daily with a multiple vitamin.

A landmark review of 38 years of scientific evidence by Harvard researchers, Dr. Robert Fletcher and Dr. Kathleen Fairfield, convinced the conservative *Journal of the American Medical Association (JAMA)* to rewrite its policy guidelines regarding the use of vitamin supplements.

In two reports, published in the June 19, 2002 edition of *JAMA*, the authors conclude that the current North American diet, while sufficient to prevent vitamin deficiency diseases (such as scurvy and pellagra), is inadequate to support the need for optimal health.

In the study, the authors examined several nutrients, including vitamins A, B_6, B_{12}, C, D, E, K, folic acid and several of the carotenoids (alpha- and beta-carotene, cryptoxanthin, zeaxanthin, lycopene and lutein). Among their conclusions, they note:

✔ folic acid, vitamin B_6 and B_{12} are required for proper homocysteine metabolism, and low levels of the vitamins are associated with increased risk of heart disease;

✔ inadequate folic acid status increases the risk of neural tube defects and some cancers;

✔ vitamin E and lycopene appear to decrease the risk of prostate cancer;

✔ vitamin D is associated with a decreased risk of osteoporosis and fracture, when taken with calcium;

✔ inadequate vitamin B_{12} is associated with anemia and neurological disorders;

✔ low levels of the carotenoids appear to increase the risk of breast, prostate and lung cancer;

✔ inadequate vitamin C is associated with increased cancer risk;

✔ low vitamin A status is associated with vision disorder and impaired immune function.

In a striking departure from *JAMA's* anti-vitamin stance of the previous twenty years, the authors conclude that, given today's diet, daily supplementation with a multiple vitamin is a prudent preventive measure against chronic disease. The researchers base their guidance on the fact that more than 80 percent of the American population does not consume anywhere near the five-per-day servings of fruits and vegetables required for optimal health.

JAMA's last comprehensive review of vitamins, conducted in the 1980s, concluded that people of normal health do not need to take a multivitamin and can meet all their nutritional needs through diet. This sudden "about-face," along with *JAMA's* public declaration that supplementation is now deemed important to your health, underscores the strength of the scientific evidence that now prevails.

The *JAMA* declaration also underscores a growing concern among nutrition experts that the current recommended intakes for vitamins and minerals are too low. The Recommended Dietary Allowances (RDAs) were originally established to prevent acute vitamin deficiency disorders; however, a growing volume of evidence supports the argument that higher levels of many vitamins and minerals are necessary to achieve optimal health.

entire amount is entered as vitamin A because the exact amount of beta-carotene cannot be determined.

Excipients

In determining the product scores, it is not feasible to evaluate the use of various fillers, additives, preservatives and coatings; nor are the questions pertaining to manufacturing, quality control, raw material sources, or purity easily addressed. These considerations, however, are important to the overall determination of product quality. In consideration of these issues, we review the top-ranking products (those that have garnered a strong product rating), in order to assess the quality practices employed in their manufacture. This information, along with a breakout of the components of the product rating, a description of the product, and details on the company, is available in Chapter 5.

Products with Phytonutrients

The bioflavonoids (including the citrus flavonoids, soy isoflavones, quercetin, quercitrin, hesperidin, rutin, bilberry extract and green tea catechins) are listed under the category of *Mixed Bioflavonoids*. The phenolic compounds (including the olive-based polyphenols and turmeric extracts) are listed under the category of *Phenolic Compounds*. The *Procyanidolic Oligomers* (PCOs)—including grape seed and pine bark extracts—form a third component. All three are listed in the *Adjusted Blended Standard*. To qualify for inclusion, product labelling information *must* include the milligram amounts of the active ingredients (i.e. 25 mg of citrus bioflavonoids, 10 mg of soy isoflavones, etc.) as opposed to the total extract or powder. If a product does not list the milligrams of the individual phytonutrient ingredients, the components are *not* included in the analysis.

Products with Ingredients Not Listed

Some products contain one or more ingredients not included in the *Blended Standard*. These products often include macro-nutritional components, such as amino acids, proteins, and carbohydrate and nucleic acid complexes. In general, these macronutrients are easily obtained through a balanced diet and, consequently, are not included. Other products contain herbal components that, while recognized for their merit, are not generally acknowledged as essential by the authorities upon which we have based our scoring criteria.

Where a product contains ingredients that are not acknowledged in the recommendations from our cited authorities, those ingredients are deemed *nonessential* for the purposes of this comparison.

Sources of Information

The formulations of the nutritional products included in this comparative guide were obtained from information provided through:
✔ product labels;
✔ product monographs;
✔ Government of Canada's Drug Product Database;[19]
✔ as available through corporate web sites and the Internet; and,
✔ through direct contact with the company.

A Cautionary Note on Toxicity

The nutrients highlighted in yellow in the product graphs have demonstrated potential retention toxicities when administered in high doses over long periods of time. These include vitamin A and iron:

Vitamin A

Ingestion of too much vitamin A can be toxic, particularly "if there are defects in storage and transport, which occurs in cirrhosis of the liver, hepatitis, protein calorie malnutrition and in children and adolescents."[20,21] Because vitamin A is fat-soluble, long-term consumption of excessive amounts through supplementation can lead to retention toxicity.

Vitamin A toxicity can be identified by the presence of fissured and dry skin, brittle nails, anorexia, irritability, fatigue and nausea.[22] Dosages greater than 10,000 IU, particularly within the first trimester of pregnancy are believed to be responsible for many of the birth defects observed in the United States.[23]

Iron

A significant proportion of our population, particularly those of northern European descent, suffer from iron overload, or haemochromatosis, a potentially fatal, genetically-linked disorder that causes the body to absorb too much iron from the diet. About one in every 250 North Americans suffer from this condition. According to Cooper (1996),[24] while the disorder is initially asymptomatic, in later stages individuals may suffer fatigue, abdominal pain, achy joints, impotence or excessive thirst and urination.

Excess iron is not excreted by the body (except during female menses) but is stored in tissues like the heart and liver. Because iron is a potent pro-oxidant and free radical generator, high serum levels can accelerate oxidative damage of cholesterol, with the consequent onset of atherosclerosis. Other risks of iron overload include an increased risk of infection, cancer,[25] and myocardial infarction (heart attack).[26]

Moreover, children and adults supplementing with high levels of ascorbic acid (vitamin C) and citric acid can increase, sometimes dramatically, their uptake of iron.[27] Consequently, caution is warranted—particularly with chewable children's tablets—if using a nutritional supplement that contains iron. Acute iron poisoning can have serious consequences.

Please keep all products containing iron out of reach of children.

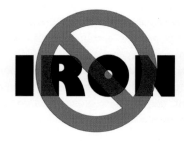

Table 3-1: Development of the Adjusted Blended Standard

Compound	Units	Dietary Reference Intakes (1) Child 4-8 yrs	Original Blended Standard	Adjusted Blended Standard (ABS)	ABS truncated @ 50% of UL	Tolerable Upper Level of Intake (UL)
Vitamins						
Vitamin A (retinol)	IU	1333	7500	2250	1500.0	3000.0
Vitamin D3 (cholecalciferol)	IU	200	350	105	105.0	2000.0
Vitamin K (phylloquinone)	µg	55	180	54	54.0	ND(2)
B-Complex Vitamins						
Biotin	µg	12	200	60	12.0	ND
Folic Acid	µg	200	400	120	120.0	400.0
Vitamin B1 (thiamin)	mg	0.6	50	15	0.6	ND
Vitamin B2 (riboflavin)	mg	0.6	43	13	0.6	ND
Vitamin B3 (niacin/niacinamide)	mg	8	75	23	7.5	15.0
Vitamin B5 (pantothenic acid)	mg	3	75	23	3.0	ND
Vitamin B6 (pyridoxine)	mg	0.6	63	19	19.0	40.0
Vitamin B12 (cobalamin)	µg	1.2	300	90	1.2	ND
Antioxidant Nutrients						
beta-Carotene	mg	ND	12500	3750	3750.0	ND
Coenzyme Q10	mg	ND	45	14	14.0	ND
alpha Lipoic Acid	mg	ND	35	11	11.0	ND
Para-Aminobenzoic Acid	mg	ND	35	11	11.0	ND
Vitamin C (ascorbic acid)	mg	25	2000	600	325.0	650.0
Vitamin E (alpha -tocopherol)	IU	10.5	500	150	150.0	450.0
Bioflavonoid Complex						
Mixed Bioflavonoids	mg	ND	555	167	167.0	ND
Phenolic Compounds (3)	mg	ND	25	8	8.0	ND
Procyanidolic Oligomers	mg	ND	75	23	23.0	ND
Glutathione Precursors						
Cysteine (n-acetyl)	mg	ND	56	17	17.0	ND
Lipid Metabolism						
Carnitine	mg	ND	750	225	225.0	ND
Choline	mg	250	59	18	18.0	1000.0
Inositol	mg	ND	125	38	38.0	ND
Lecithin	mg	ND	350	105	105.0	ND
Minerals						
Boron	mg	ND	3	1	1.0	6.0
Calcium	mg	800	800	240	240.0	2500.0
Chromium	µg	15	275	83	15.0	ND
Copper	mg	0.44	2	1	1.0	3.0
Iodine	µg	90	100	30	30.0	300.0
Iron	mg	10	23	7	7.0	40.0
Magnesium (4)	mg	130	450	135	110.0	110.0
Manganese	mg	1.5	7	2	1.5	3.0
Molybdenum	µg	22	63	19	19.0	600.0
Potassium	mg	3,800	300	90	90.0	ND
Selenium	µg	30	150	45	45.0	150.0
Silicon	mg	ND	8	2	2.0	ND
Vanadium	µg	ND	75	23	23.0	ND
Zinc	mg	5	23	7	6.0	12.0

(1) Includes total daily intake from all sources
(2) ND implies not determined
(3) Recommended level of phenolic acids adapted from: Visioli F, et al. Atherosclerosis. 1995;117:25-32.
(4) Magnesium intake from a pharmacological agent only and does not include intake from food and water.

Dietary Reference Intakes and Tolerable Upper Limits data cited from:
Dietary Reference Intakes, Food and Nutrition Board, Institute of Medicine, National Academies. Available at:
http://www.iom.edu/ Accessed: August 26,2004.

Details of the original Blended Standard are available in: MacWilliam L, Comparative Guide to Nutritional Supplements (3rd edition).
Northern Dimensions Publishing, Vernon, British Columbia, 2003, pp 62-63.

mins and herbs, and the issue of regulatory control needed to ensure safety has become a growing concern.

For this reason, the Government of Canada has created a new regulatory environment for vitamins, minerals and herbal products. Since January 2004, all Canadian nutritional supplements fall under the purview of the new Natural Health Products Directorate (NHPD).

All businesses in Canada that wish to manufacture or import a natural health product must have a license to do so. The license ensures that the manufacturer follows acceptable good manufacturing practices. Canada's Natural Health Products Regulations also require manufacturers to obtain a product license before they can sell or distribute a natural health product.

Previous to 2004, any manufacturer selling a vitamin product in Canada was required to obtain a Drug Identity Number (DIN), signifying that the product met acceptable pharmaceutical standards for manufacture. Today, manufacturers of nutritional supplements must apply for a NHPD product number (NPN). Similar to the old DIN application, the process involves evaluation for compliance with acceptable manufacturing and labelling standards. The presence of an NPN or DIN ensures that a product meets federally-mandated quality and safety standards. All natural health products sold in Canada must prominently display the product number on the label.

Profiling the Top-rated Products

In Chapter 5, we profile the top products evaluated in this comparative guide. We attempt to provide as much information as we can obtain on the standards of manufacturing employed by the leading nutritional manufacturers that we have identified. Because U.S. standards are so relaxed—and there is no need for public disclosure of the information—it is sometimes difficult to assess the level of manufacturing and product quality. Some companies are not particularly forthcoming with such information. That said, industry leaders who voluntarily comply with pharmaceutical GMPs are more than happy to provide details on their manufacturing and product quality practices.

In the U.S., look for companies that adopt pharmaceutical (USP) GMPs and product quality standards.

In Canada, a DIN (now being phased out) or NPN identity number is your assurance that the product has met rigorous, federally-mandated standards. Remember that no nutritional

product can be legally sold in Canada without one of these Health Canada designations.

Along with our *Final Product Scores*, indication that the product meets pharmaceutical GMPs and product quality standards (United States), or bears an NPN or DIN designation (Canada), will ensure that you have selected a quality product.

Product Quality Checklist

Here's a quick do-it-yourself checklist to help you evaluate whether a particular product is worthy of consideration. Ask yourself these questions:

1. Is the product delivered in a multiple dose? A once-a-day tablet simply cannot provide the levels of potency needed for optimal nutrition without being too large to swallow.
2. Are the potency levels of the ingredients high enough to provide optimal daily nutritional intake *without* compromising safety?
3. Are the ingredients provided in the most bioavailable form? Mineral salts are not as well absorbed as chelated minerals or minerals bound to an organic carrier.
4. Is the safety profile of each ingredient thoroughly researched and evaluated?
5. Does the company meet United States (pharmaceutical-grade) and Canadian (Natural Health Product-grade) Good Manufacturing Processes (GMPs)?
6. Is the product formulated to meet pharmaceutical-grade standards for disintegration and dissolution?
7. Is the product potency guaranteed for a specified shelf life?
8. Is the product manufactured in-house, or is it contracted out to the lowest bidder?
9. Is the product independently tested and guaranteed for potency and safety?
10. Does the product contain levels of pre-formed vitamin A and iron (nutrients known to have potential retention toxicities) that are well below their tolerable upper limits of intake (ULs)? Products that are free of iron and deliver their vitamin A from beta-carotene are preferable.

If the product meets all of these criteria, you know that you have a nutritional supplement of exceptional quality. If it doesn't, keep looking—or consider one of the top products highlighted in this guide.

1. Center for Food Safety and Applied Nutrition. "Overview of Dietary Supplements" *U.S Food and Drug Administration,* http://www.cfsan.fda.gov/~dms/ds-oview.html#regulate, 2001

**The way to gain a good reputation
is to endeavor to be what you desire to appear.**

—*Socrates (469 BC - 399 BC)*

CHAPTER FIVE

TOP PRODUCTS OVERALL

Leaders in the Nutritional Supplement Marketplace

We examined over 250 Canadian and American nutritional products in writing this Comparative Guide. From this, 160 qualifying products, representing the best in the line-up of some 120 companies, were further evaluated and compared to the selected nutritional standards, according to nutrient content and daily intake. Graphical comparisons were completed on one hundred and thirty-seven (137) finalists, representing the top-rated product(s) from each manufacturer. Some companies have more than one product represented if they market in both Canada and the United States.

This chapter provides detailed information on the top fifteen scoring nutritional products and the companies that manufacture or distribute them. A four- to five-star rating is evidence that the product scored exceptionally well against our 14 assessment criteria. Fewer than 5 percent of the 250 products examined achieved a score of four stars; and only 1.2 percent achieved a five-star rating.

Table 5-1 (below) shows the top-scoring products and their ratings on our five-star scale. For a complete listing of all products and their *Final Product Scores*, please refer to Appendices A and B.

Table 5-1: Top 15 Products

Rank	Product Name	Country	Star Rating
1	*Douglas Laboratories Vita-Big-Kids*	🇺🇸	★★★★★
2	*USANA Health Sciences Usanimals*	🇨🇦	★★★★★
3	*USANA Health Sciences Usanimals*	🇺🇸	★★★★★
4	*Douglas Laboratories Basic Preventive Junior*	🇺🇸	★★★★☆
5	*SISU Mini-Vits*	🇨🇦	★★★★☆
6	*ProThera VitaTab Chewable*	🇺🇸	★★★★☆
7	*SuperNutrition Perfect Kids*	🇺🇸	★★★★☆
8	*Douglas Laboratories Children's Essentials*	🇺🇸	★★★★☆
9	*Pharmanex Jungamals*	🇺🇸	★★★★☆
10	*Source Naturals Mega-Kid Multiple*	🇺🇸	★★★★☆
11	*DaVinci Laboratories Omni Jr.*	🇺🇸	★★★★☆
12	*Vitamin Research Products Kids Essentials*	🇺🇸	★★★★☆
13	*SISU Mini-Vits*	🇺🇸	★★★★☆
14	*Natural Factors Big Friends*	🇨🇦	★★★★☆
15	*Natural Factors Learning Factors*	🇨🇦	★★★★☆

Douglas Laboratories

600 Boyce Road, Pittsburgh, Pennsylvania, USA 15205

Phone: 412-494-0122 Toll-free (US): 888-368-4522 (CA) 866-856-9954

Fax: 412-494-0155

Web Site: www.douglaslabs.com

Availability: Retail, Online

Ownership: Private

General Information: Under the direction of President Jeffry Lioon and CEO Douglas Lioon, the company has a staff of over 250 laboratory employees. With three in-house laboratories, outfitted with the latest high-tech analytical equipment, the company produces nearly 1000 products that meet pharmaceutical GMPs, USP product quality standards and other worldwide standards, including ISO 9001 and ISO 17025. The company also provides custom formulations, private labelling and packaging for those customers who wish to market their own brand of natural products.

Philosophy: The company is committed to raising the standard for nutrition and wellness.

Quality: Products meet, and often exceed, USP standards. The facility is routinely inspected by the FDA and international representatives. Products are approved by Health Canada and the Commission of the European Communities. Written procedures for each aspect of production adhere to strict quality-control standards. Testing and sampling of all raw materials are conducted and records kept of each component and the quantity used in every batch of product. Microbiological testing on all products ensures that they meet or exceed USP microbial-limit requirements. Finished products are tested to ensure USP standards for dissolution tests and pH, and product potency is verified with High Pressure Liquid Chromatography.

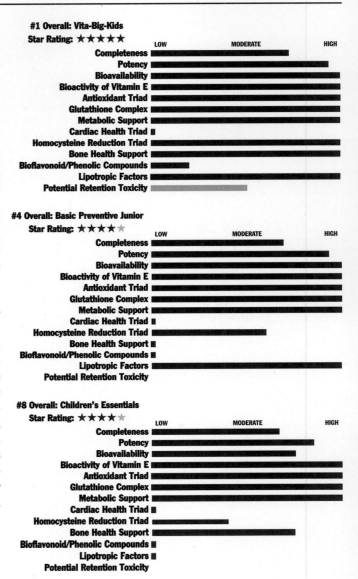

#1 Overall: Vita-Big-Kids
Star Rating: ★★★★★

#4 Overall: Basic Preventive Junior
Star Rating: ★★★★☆

#8 Overall: Children's Essentials
Star Rating: ★★★★☆

USANA Health Sciences

3838 West Parkway Blvd., Salt Lake City, Utah, USA 84120

Phone: 801-954-7100

Order Line: 888-950-9595

Web Site (corporate): www.usanahealthsciences.com

Web Site (product): www.usana-nutritionals.com

Availability: Online, Direct Sales

Ownership: Publicly traded on NASDAQ as USNA

General Information: Microbiologist and immunologist Dr. Myron Wentz established USANA Health Sciences in 1992 to create products that provide antioxidant protection and overall cellular nutrition for the body. The primary focus of the company is to develop and market scientifically advanced nutritional products to help prevent degenerative disease and promote optimal health. USANA products are sold directly to Preferred Customers and Associates in the United States, Canada, Australia, New Zealand, the United Kingdom, the Netherlands, Hong Kong, Japan, Taiwan and Singapore. The company was featured in a December 2002 CBS Marketwatch report as the #3 performing U.S. stock in that year. USANA has selected the Children's Hunger Fund as its charitable organization of choice, and helps the organization in its mission of providing basic nutrition for children suffering from malnourishment and hunger.

Philosophy: The Company's Mission Statement is "to develop and provide the highest quality, science-based health products, distributed internationally through Network Marketing, creating a rewarding financial opportunity for our Independent Associates, shareholders and employees."

Quality: The Company voluntarily meets Good Manufacturing Practices (GMPs) for pharmaceutical-grade products, eclipsing the standards followed by most nutritional product manufacturers. Raw ingredients are quarantined until tested and quality control tests are conducted on the products during manufacturing. Written quality assurance criteria track all testing and evaluation from raw materials to finished product. Products are laboratory tested and guaranteed to meet USP specifications for quality, potency and disintegration, where applicable. The company is registered with the FDA as a pharmaceutical manufacturer.

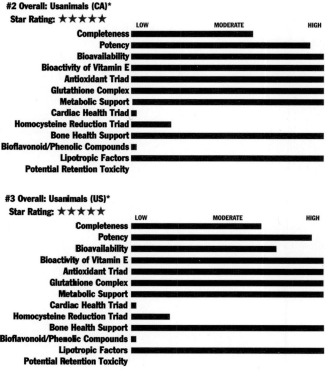

Product ratings differ due to regulatory differences between the countries. The Canadian component does not consider either vitamin K or boron, as these nutrients have not, until recently, been allowed in Canadian nutritional products.

SISU

104A-3430 Brighton Ave., Burnaby, BC, Canada V5A 3H4

Phone: 604-420-6610 Toll-free 800-663-4163

Fax: 604-420-4892 Toll-free 888-420-6640

Web Site: www.sisu.com

Availability: Retail

Ownership: Private

General Information: Convinced through research, education, and experience that people could stay healthy longer and recover from illness more rapidly through the prudent use of well-formulated vitamins and supplements, pharmacist Harlan Lahti founded SISU. His goal was to create and produce formulas that would meet the exacting standards of the Canadian government, rise even higher to satisfy the requirements of physicians, and provide discerning consumers with the very best supplements possible. The word "sisu" can be loosely translated from Finnish as "strength and stubborn determination" combined with "stamina and courage"—especially when overcoming obstacles. SISU is dedicated to wellness, helping active and health-conscious consumers manage their health and wellness needs.

Philosophy: The company's mission is to be the leader in providing high quality alternative health products and services that substantially improve the wellness in the community.

Quality: No information on specific manufacturing processes is available. Canadian manufactuers must, by law, meet requirements for Good Manufacturing Practices and finished product quality stipulated by Health Canada's new Natural Health Products Directorate.

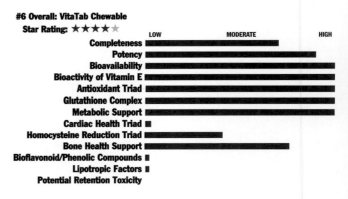

ProThera Inc.

4133 Mohr Avenue, Suite I, Pleasanton, CA, USA 94566

Phone: 1-888-488-2488, 925-484-5636

Fax: 925-484-9055

Web Site: www.protherainc.com

Availability: Medical professionals

Ownership: Private

General Information: ProThera, Inc. manufactures a comprehensive line of nutraceutical products for exclusive distribution by healthcare professionals. Products are designed for medical applications based on 45 years of combined formulation experience by the company's founders, Dennis Meiss, Ph.D. and Janet Ralston, B.S., working in close association with an advisory board of medical consultants with extensive clinical experience in nutritional medicine. A coordinated group of multinutrient products with focused clinical applications forms the core of the ProThera product line, with emphasis given to avoiding nutrient redundancy, maintaining cost-effectiveness, and encouraging patient compliance.

Philosophy: ProThera dietary supplements are carefully designed to maximize the synergism between nutrients.

Quality: ProThera nutraceuticals are produced in licensed manufacturing facilities that strictly adhere to current Good Manufacturing Practices (cGMPs). The manufacturing facility is approved to manufacture a drug product by the FDA and by governmental agencies in California, the United Kingdom, the European Community (EC) and Australia. Current GMPs and written standard operating procedures (SOPs) are strictly followed through all stages of production to produce products that meet or exceed United States Pharmacopeia (USP) standards. Purity and potency of selected raw materials are verified through independent testing laboratories by raw material vendors and ProThera, Inc. All incoming raw materials undergo quarantine, inspection, and evaluation.

---

* *Product ratings differ due to regulatory differences between the countries. The Canadian component does not consider either vitamin K or boron, as these nutrients have not, until recently, been allowed in Canadian nutritional products.*

SuperNutrition

1925 Brush Street, Oakland, California, USA 94612

Phone: 800-262-2116

Fax: 510-446-7994

Web Site: www.supernutritionusa.com

Availability: Online, Retail

Ownership: Private, family owned and operated

General Information: SuperNutrition was founded in 1977 by Patrick Mooney, his son, Michael Mooney, and Sandra Barros, to evaluate and disseminate information about the new breakthroughs in nutritional biochemistry and their effects on health. Located in San Francisco for 24 years, SuperNutrition recently moved across the San Francisco Bay to Oakland California. The company specializes in orthomolecular daily multivitamin formulas. Products are available at Health and Natural Food Stores across the USA.

Philosophy: Corporate Mission Statement not available.

Quality: All organic ingredients are organically grown and processed in accordance with the California Organic Foods Act of 1990. Most products are hypoallergenic and contain no yeast, wheat, gluten, buckwheat, pollen, dairy, corn or soy residues or any hidden additives. No specific information was available at the time of writing on whether the company voluntarily adopts pharmaceutical GMPs or product quality standards (FDA standards for nutritional supplements require only food-grade rather than pharmaceutical-grade GMPs).

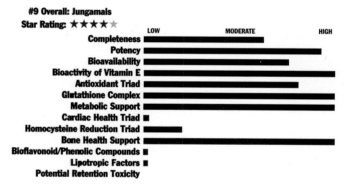

Pharmanex

75 West Center, Provo, Utah, USA 84601

Phone: 800-487-1000

Fax: 800-487-8000

Web Site: www.pharmanexusa.com

Availability: Online, Direct Sales

Ownership: Subsidiary of Nu Skin Enterprises, which is publicly traded on New York Stock Exchange (NYSE: NUS)

General Information: Pharmanex, a Nu Skin Enterprises' company, is a leader in the research and development of phyto-pharmaceutical and nutritional products. The company is headquartered in Provo, Utah. Pharmanex's annual world-wide sales have reached nearly $400 million throughout the United States, Asia and Europe. In 1998, Pharmanex became a fully owned subsidiary of Nu Skin Enterprises (NSE). NSE boasts more than a decade of innovation, financial stability and leadership, and is now one of the largest direct-selling companies in the world.

Philosophy: Under the leadership of Dr. Joseph Chang, Pharmanex employees are highly committed to accomplishing the company's mission: to help people achieve more healthy and productive lives.

Quality: Pharmanex uses a proprietary quality control system it calls "6S." By applying this process, Pharmanex has consistently met or exceeded the Good Manufacturing Practices (GMPs) set by the FDA for this product category (FDA standards for nutritional supplements require only food-grade rather than pharmaceutical-grade GMPs). Pharmanex indicates that pharmaceutical-grade tests are used for the presence of microbes, toxins, and heavy metals for all products.

Source Naturals

19 Janis Way, Scotts Valley, California, USA 95066

Phone: 831-438-1144 Toll-free: 800-815-2333

Fax: 831-438-7410

Web Site: www.sourcenaturals.com

Availability: Online, Retail

Ownership: Private, Threshold Enterprises Ltd.

General Information: Source Naturals was founded by CEO Ira Goldberg, in 1982. With the introduction of its Wellness Formula® for natural immune support, Source Naturals became an early pioneer in the use of integrated formulations, consisting of vitamins, minerals, herbs, amino acids, and nutraceuticals.

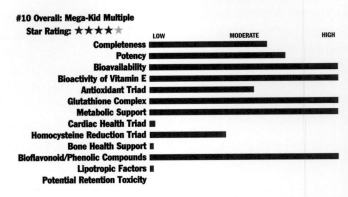

Today, Source Naturals manufactures a line of comprehensive products using its proprietary Bio-Aligned Formulas,™ designed to help bring the power of "alignment" to the body by evaluating the root causes of body system imbalances, and then providing targeted nutrition. Source Naturals' line of more than 400 products reflects the latest advances in nutritional research, with a comprehensive selection of nutrients in their highest quality and most bioavailable forms. Products are sold through storefront retailers throughout the United States and through online retailers in the U.S. and Europe.

Philosophy: Source Naturals recognizes that supplementation is only one part of optimum health: this requires an overall program that encompasses a healthy diet, sufficient exercise and relaxation, good sleeping habits, and lots more.

Quality: Raw materials are evaluated for certificate of analysis and finished products are "inspected to ensure that they meet a long list of Acceptable Quality Limits, based on industry standards and our own exacting requirements." The company seeks to minimize excipients in its products and to use the most natural sources available. No specific information was available at the time of writing on whether the company voluntarily adopts pharmaceutical GMPs or product quality standards (FDA standards for nutritional supplements require only food-grade rather than pharmaceutical-grade GMPs).

DaVinci Laboratories of Vermont

20 New England Drive Essex Junction, Vermont 05453

Phone: U.S. & Canada Toll Free: 1-800-325-1776

Fax: 1-802-878-0549

Web Site: www.davincilabs.com

Availability: Medical Professionals, Online

Ownership: Information unavailable at the time of writing.

General Information: For over 25 years, DaVinci Laboratories of Vermont has been a leader in nutritional research and product development, selling exclusively to healthcare professionals worldwide. DaVinci labs offers a full range of specialty products, such as immune system support supplements, joint and connec-

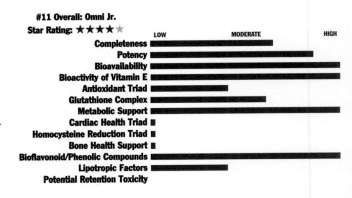

tive tissue formulas, eye, prostate, and menopause support supplements as well as a complete line of high potency multiple vitamin/mineral formulas that are age and gender specific.

Philosophy: Mission statement not available.

Quality: Raw materials used in the company's products are as natural as possible and are guaranteed to contain no artificial flavorings, preservatives, colors, sweeteners or other foreign agents unless otherwise stated on the label. Each lot of tablets or capsules is carefully assayed to be sure they meet DaVinci's product quality specifications. No specific information was available at the time of writing on whether the company voluntarily adopts pharmaceutical GMPs or product quality standards (FDA standards for nutritional supplements require only food-grade rather than pharmaceutical-grade GMPs).

Vitamin Research Products

3579 Highway 50 East, Carson City, NV 89701
Phone: 800-877-2447 Int'l: 775-884-8210
Order Line: 775-884-1300
Fax: 775-884-1331
Web Site: www.vrp.com
Availability: Online
Ownership: Private

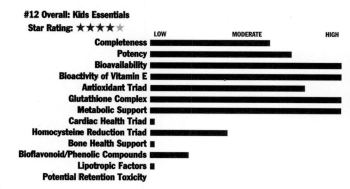

General Information: Vitamin Research Products was born in 1979, when a small group of scientists, responding to the need for pharmaceutically pure high potency antioxidant formulations, decided to create their own company and develop their own special formulas. Today, Vitamin Research Products manufactures and distributes more than 450 supplements. Formulas are based on the latest clinical research and use pharmaceutical-quality ingredients. The company also provides online consultations with nutritional consultants.

Philosophy: The company is committed to making the world's finest nutritional formulas, underscored by the choice to provide most formulas in capsules, not tablets, which the company believes maximizes nutrient content, absorption and potency.

Quality: Vitamin Research Products uses USP-grade ingredients in their formulations, with quality verification through high-pressure liquid chromatography (HPLC). No specific information was available at the time of writing on whether the company voluntarily adopts pharmaceutical GMPs or product quality standards (FDA standards for nutritional supplements require only food-grade rather than pharmaceutical-grade GMPs).

Natural Factors Nutritional Products Ltd.

1550 United Boulevard, Coquitlam, BC, Canada V3K 6Y7
Phone: 604-777-1757 Toll-free 800-663-8900
Fax: 604-420-0772 Toll-free 800-663-2115
Web Site: www.naturalfactors.com
Availability: Retail (health food stores)
Ownership: Private.

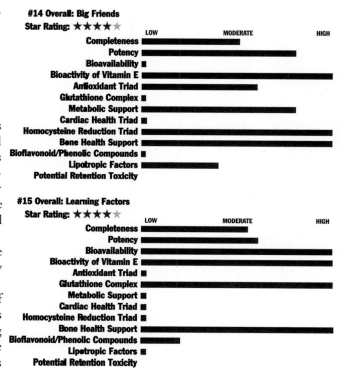

General Information: For more than 50 years, the Gahler family has been producing and distributing quality products for the natural health consumer. Roland Gahler has been leading Natural Factors for the past few decades, adding modern technological improvements and investing in scientific research that contributes to greater reliability and effectiveness of the company's natural products. The product line reflects the company's holistic approach to personal health.

Philosophy: The company's goal is to deliver products which marry the wisdom of ancient herbal physicians and the science of exciting, new clinical research to maximize the health of its customers.

Quality: Natural Factors' products undergo rigorous testing at all levels of the production process in accordance with United States Pharmacopoeia (USP) guidelines. Manufacturing is done according to Good Manufacturing Practices (GMP) guidelines mandated by the Health Protection Branch (HPB) of Health Canada. Factors Laboratories also follows Good Laboratory Practices (GLP) guidelines. Natural Factors' Quality Control department and laboratory are involved in every step of its product development, including pre-production and post-production product testing.

CHAPTER SIX

GRAPHICAL COMPARISONS

This section provides the reader
with an in-depth look at:

■ Graphical comparisons of 137 products
    from Canadian and U.S. companies
■ Top-rated products from each company
■ All products compared to the
    Adjusted Blended Standard

*One hundred thirty-seven graphical comparisons of the top
performing multi-vitamin and mineral products from over one
hundred U.S. and Canadian companies are presented. Relative
scores, based on a five-star scale are provided. Each product is
graphically compared to the selected reference standard, based
on the relative product scores.*

Graphical Comparisons to the Adjusted Blended Standard

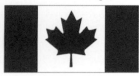

Canadian Product Comparisons

Canadian products do not include boron or vitamin K, and ratings have been adjusted accordingly. Previously prohibited in Canada, these nutrients will be evaluated by the new Natural Health Products Directorate.

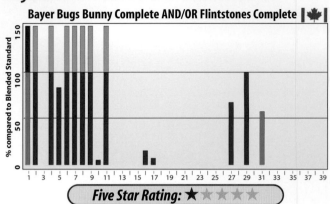

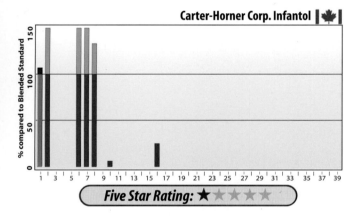

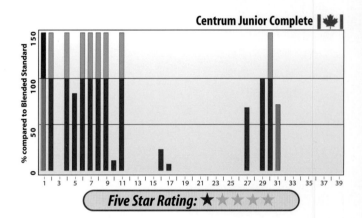

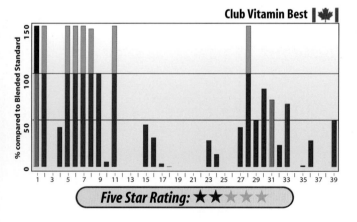

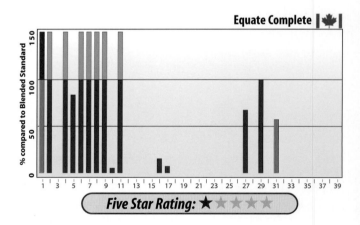

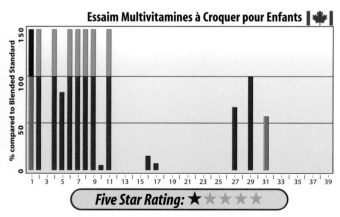

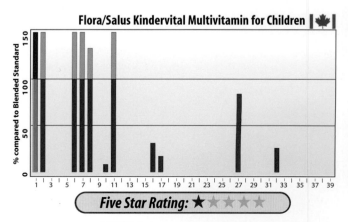

Graphical Comparisons to the Adjusted Blended Standard

Adjusted Blended Standard

#	Nutrient	Amount	#	Nutrient	Amount
1	Vitamin A	1500.0 IU	21	n-Acetyl-l-Cysteine	17.0 mg
2	Vitamin D3	105.0 IU	22	l-Carnitine	225.0 mg
3	Vitamin K*	54.0 ug	23	Choline	18.0 mg
4	Biotin	12.0 ug	24	Inositol	38.0 mg
5	Folic Acid	120.0 ug	25	Lecithin	105.0 mg
6	Vitamin B₁	0.6 mg	26	Boron*	1.0 mg
7	Vitamin B₂	0.6 mg	27	Calcium	240.0 mg
8	Vitamin B₃ complex	7.5 mg	28	Chromium	15.0 ug
9	Vitamin B₅	3.0 mg	29	Copper	1.0 mg
10	Vitamin B₆	19.0 mg	30	Iodine	30.0 ug
11	Vitamin B₁₂	1.2 ug	31	Iron	7.0 mg
12	beta-Carotene	3750.0 IU	32	Magnesium	110.0 mg
13	Coenzyme Q₁₀	14.0 mg	33	Manganese	1.5 mg
14	Lipoic Acid	11.0 mg	34	Molybdenum	19.0 ug
15	Para-Aminobenzoic Acid	11.0 mg	35	Potassium	90.0 mg
16	Vitamin C	325.0 mg	36	Selenium	45.0 ug
17	Vitamin E	150.0 IU	37	Silicon	2.0 mg
18	Bioflavonoids (mixed)	167.0 mg	38	Vanadium	23.0 ug
19	Phenolic compounds	8.0 mg	39	Zinc	6.0 mg
20	Procyanidolic Oligomers	23.0 mg		* Not Available in Canadian Products	

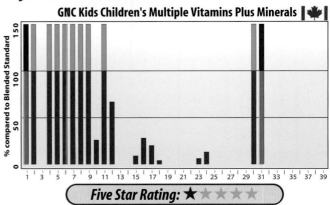

GNC Kids Children's Multiple Vitamins Plus Minerals

Five Star Rating: ★ ☆ ☆ ☆ ☆

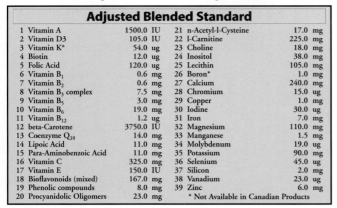

Goldshield Elite Herbal Supplements Kid's Stuff

Five Star Rating: ★ ☆ ☆ ☆ ☆

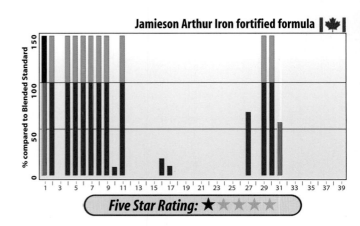

Jamieson Arthur Iron fortified formula

Five Star Rating: ★ ☆ ☆ ☆ ☆

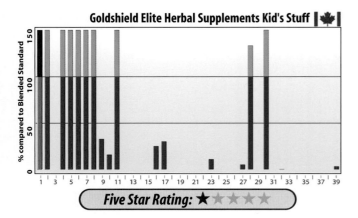

Kaire Essentials Children's Chewables

Five Star Rating: ★ ☆ ☆ ☆ ☆

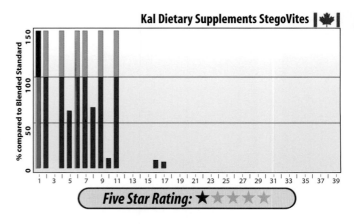

Kal Dietary Supplements StegoVites

Five Star Rating: ★ ☆ ☆ ☆ ☆

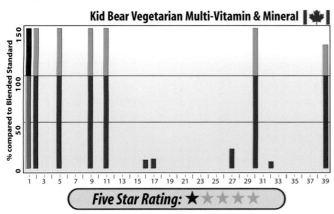

Kid Bear Vegetarian Multi-Vitamin & Mineral

Five Star Rating: ★ ☆ ☆ ☆ ☆

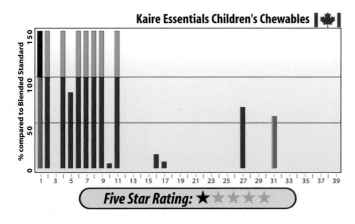

Kirkland Signature Children's Chewable MultiVitamin

Five Star Rating: ★ ☆ ☆ ☆ ☆

Graphical Comparisons to the Adjusted Blended Standard

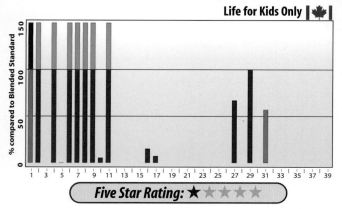

Life for Kids Only 🍁

Five Star Rating: ★ ☆ ☆ ☆ ☆

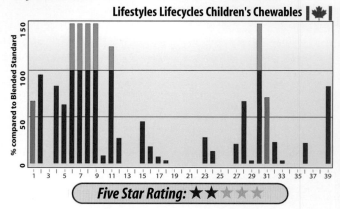

Lifestyles Lifecycles Children's Chewables 🍁

Five Star Rating: ★ ★ ☆ ☆ ☆

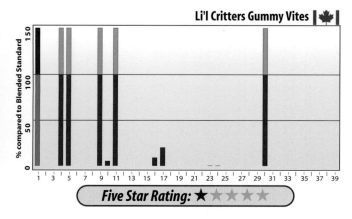

Li'l Critters Gummy Vites 🍁

Five Star Rating: ★ ☆ ☆ ☆ ☆

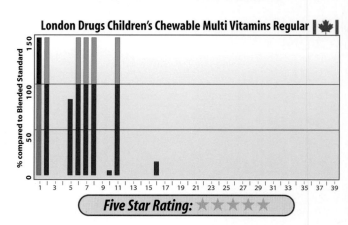

London Drugs Children's Chewable Multi Vitamins Regular 🍁

Five Star Rating: ☆ ☆ ☆ ☆ ☆

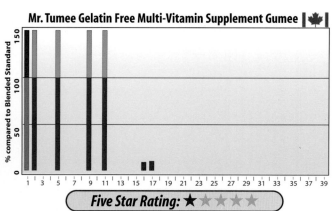

Mr. Tumee Gelatin Free Multi-Vitamin Supplement Gumee 🍁

Five Star Rating: ★ ☆ ☆ ☆ ☆

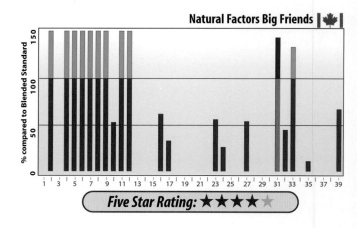

Natural Factors Big Friends 🍁

Five Star Rating: ★ ★ ★ ★ ☆

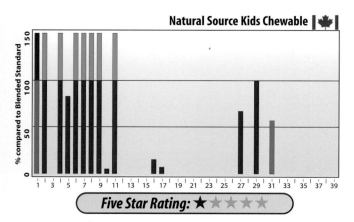

Natural Source Kids Chewable 🍁

Five Star Rating: ★ ☆ ☆ ☆ ☆

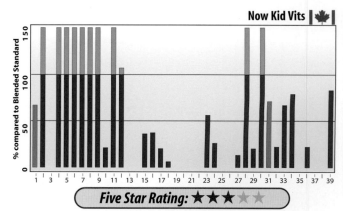

Now Kid Vits 🍁

Five Star Rating: ★ ★ ★ ☆ ☆

Graphical Comparisons to the Adjusted Blended Standard

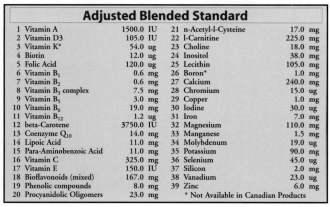

Adjusted Blended Standard

1	Vitamin A	1500.0 IU	21	n-Acetyl-l-Cysteine	17.0 mg
2	Vitamin D3	105.0 IU	22	l-Carnitine	225.0 mg
3	Vitamin K*	54.0 ug	23	Choline	18.0 mg
4	Biotin	12.0 ug	24	Inositol	38.0 mg
5	Folic Acid	120.0 ug	25	Lecithin	105.0 mg
6	Vitamin B_1	0.6 mg	26	Boron*	1.0 mg
7	Vitamin B_2	0.6 mg	27	Calcium	240.0 mg
8	Vitamin B_3 complex	7.5 mg	28	Chromium	15.0 ug
9	Vitamin B_5	3.0 mg	29	Copper	1.0 mg
10	Vitamin B_6	19.0 mg	30	Iodine	30.0 ug
11	Vitamin B_{12}	1.2 ug	31	Iron	7.0 mg
12	beta-Carotene	3750.0 IU	32	Magnesium	110.0 mg
13	Coenzyme Q_{10}	14.0 mg	33	Manganese	1.5 mg
14	Lipoic Acid	11.0 mg	34	Molybdenum	19.0 ug
15	Para-Aminobenzoic Acid	11.0 mg	35	Potassium	90.0 mg
16	Vitamin C	325.0 mg	36	Selenium	45.0 ug
17	Vitamin E	150.0 IU	37	Silicon	2.0 mg
18	Bioflavonoids (mixed)	167.0 mg	38	Vanadium	23.0 ug
19	Phenolic compounds	8.0 mg	39	Zinc	6.0 mg
20	Procyanidolic Oligomers	23.0 mg		* Not Available in Canadian Products	

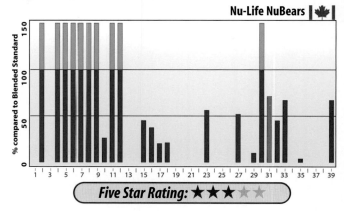

Nu-Life NuBears

Five Star Rating: ★★★☆☆

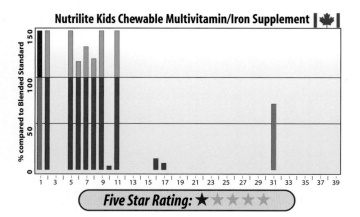

Nutrilite Kids Chewable Multivitamin/Iron Supplement

Five Star Rating: ★☆☆☆☆

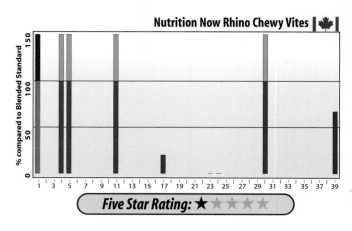

Nutrition Now Rhino Chewy Vites

Five Star Rating: ★☆☆☆☆

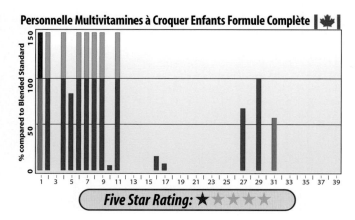

Personnelle Multivitamines à Croquer Enfants Formule Complète

Five Star Rating: ★☆☆☆☆

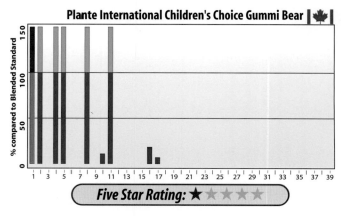

Plante International Children's Choice Gummi Bear

Five Star Rating: ★☆☆☆☆

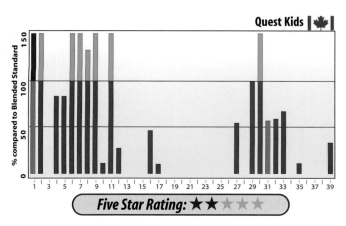

Quest Kids

Five Star Rating: ★★☆☆☆

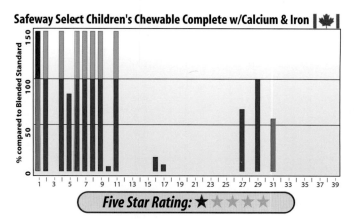

Safeway Select Children's Chewable Complete w/Calcium & Iron

Five Star Rating: ★☆☆☆☆

Graphical Comparisons to the Adjusted Blended Standard

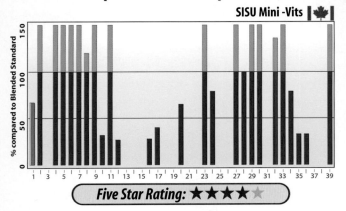

SISU Mini-Vits 🍁

Five Star Rating: ★★★★☆

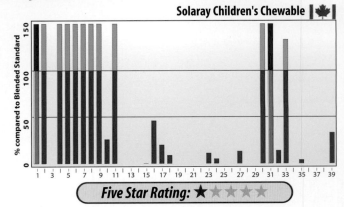

Solaray Children's Chewable 🍁

Five Star Rating: ★☆☆☆☆

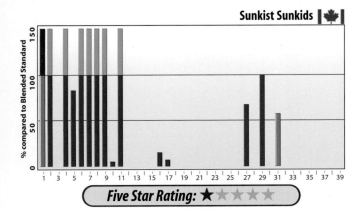

Sunkist Sunkids 🍁

Five Star Rating: ★☆☆☆☆

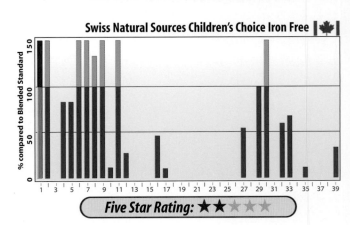

Swiss Natural Sources Children's Choice Iron Free 🍁

Five Star Rating: ★★☆☆☆

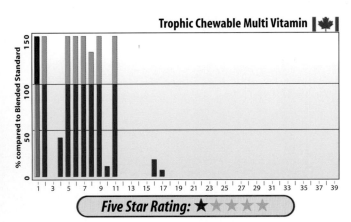

Trophic Chewable Multi Vitamin 🍁

Five Star Rating: ★☆☆☆☆

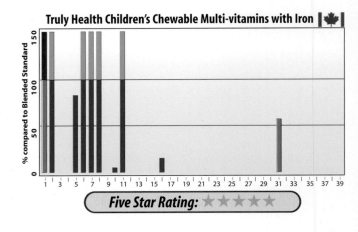

Truly Health Children's Chewable Multi-vitamins with Iron 🍁

Five Star Rating: ☆☆☆☆☆

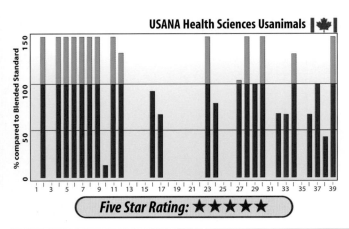

USANA Health Sciences Usanimals 🍁

Five Star Rating: ★★★★★

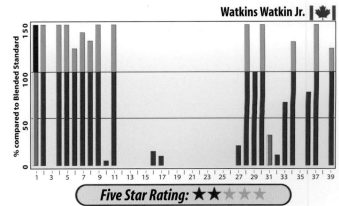

Watkins Watkin Jr. 🍁

Five Star Rating: ★★☆☆☆

Graphical Comparisons to the Adjusted Blended Standard

Adjusted Blended Standard

1	Vitamin A	1500.0	IU	21	n-Acetyl-l-Cysteine	17.0	mg
2	Vitamin D3	105.0	IU	22	l-Carnitine	225.0	mg
3	Vitamin K*	54.0	ug	23	Choline	18.0	mg
4	Biotin	12.0	ug	24	Inositol	38.0	mg
5	Folic Acid	120.0	ug	25	Lecithin	105.0	mg
6	Vitamin B$_1$	0.6	mg	26	Boron*	1.0	mg
7	Vitamin B$_2$	0.6	mg	27	Calcium	240.0	mg
8	Vitamin B$_3$ complex	7.5	mg	28	Chromium	15.0	ug
9	Vitamin B$_5$	3.0	mg	29	Copper	1.0	mg
10	Vitamin B$_6$	19.0	mg	30	Iodine	30.0	ug
11	Vitamin B$_{12}$	1.2	ug	31	Iron	7.0	mg
12	beta-Carotene	3750.0	IU	32	Magnesium	110.0	mg
13	Coenzyme Q$_{10}$	14.0	mg	33	Manganese	1.5	mg
14	Lipoic Acid	11.0	mg	34	Molybdenum	19.0	ug
15	Para-Aminobenzoic Acid	11.0	mg	35	Potassium	90.0	mg
16	Vitamin C	325.0	mg	36	Selenium	45.0	ug
17	Vitamin E	150.0	IU	37	Silicon	2.0	mg
18	Bioflavonoids (mixed)	167.0	mg	38	Vanadium	23.0	ug
19	Phenolic compounds	8.0	mg	39	Zinc	6.0	mg
20	Procyanidolic Oligomers	23.0	mg		* Not Available in Canadian Products		

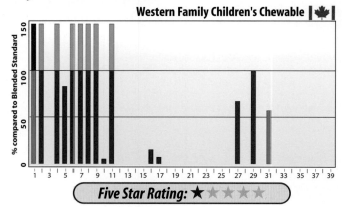

Western Family Children's Chewable

Five Star Rating: ★ ☆ ☆ ☆ ☆

Graphical Comparisons to the Adjusted Blended Standard

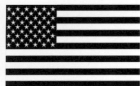

United States Product Comparisons

U.S. products may include boron and vitamin K. Ratings have been adjusted accordingly. One or both of these nutrients figure in the Completeness, Potency, Bioavailability and Bone Health criteria.

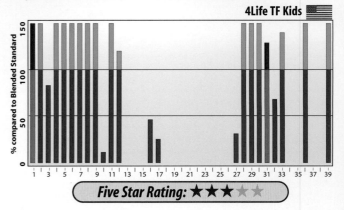

4Life TF Kids

Five Star Rating: ★★★☆☆

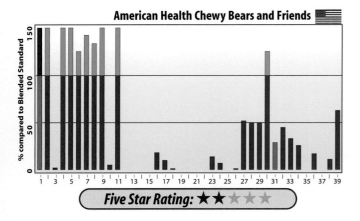

21st CENTURY Zoo Friends Complete

Five Star Rating: ★☆☆☆☆

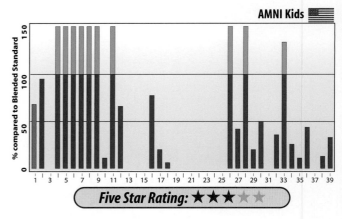

Allergy Research Group Children's Multi-Vi-Min

Five Star Rating: ★★★☆☆

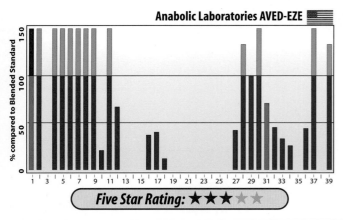

American Health Chewy Bears and Friends

Five Star Rating: ★★☆☆☆

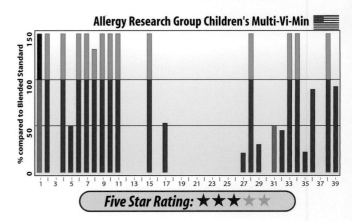

AMNI Kids

Five Star Rating: ★★★☆☆

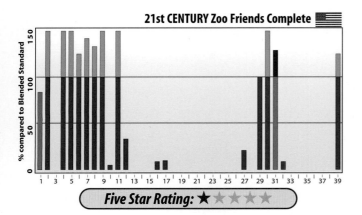

Anabolic Laboratories AVED-EZE

Five Star Rating: ★★★☆☆

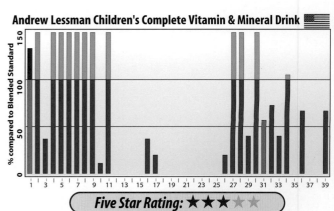

Andrew Lessman Children's Complete Vitamin & Mineral Drink

Five Star Rating: ★★★☆☆

Graphical Comparisons to the Adjusted Blended Standard

Adjusted Blended Standard

#	Nutrient	Amount	Unit	#	Nutrient	Amount	Unit
1	Vitamin A	1500.0	IU	21	n-Acetyl-l-Cysteine	17.0	mg
2	Vitamin D3	105.0	IU	22	l-Carnitine	225.0	mg
3	Vitamin K*	54.0	ug	23	Choline	18.0	mg
4	Biotin	12.0	ug	24	Inositol	38.0	mg
5	Folic Acid	120.0	ug	25	Lecithin	105.0	mg
6	Vitamin B_1	0.6	mg	26	Boron*	1.0	mg
7	Vitamin B_2	0.6	mg	27	Calcium	240.0	mg
8	Vitamin B_3 complex	7.5	mg	28	Chromium	15.0	ug
9	Vitamin B_5	3.0	mg	29	Copper	1.0	mg
10	Vitamin B_6	19.0	mg	30	Iodine	30.0	ug
11	Vitamin B_{12}	1.2	ug	31	Iron	7.0	mg
12	beta-Carotene	3750.0	IU	32	Magnesium	110.0	mg
13	Coenzyme Q_{10}	14.0	mg	33	Manganese	1.5	mg
14	Lipoic Acid	11.0	mg	34	Molybdenum	19.0	ug
15	Para-Aminobenzoic Acid	11.0	mg	35	Potassium	90.0	mg
16	Vitamin C	325.0	mg	36	Selenium	45.0	ug
17	Vitamin E	150.0	IU	37	Silicon	2.0	mg
18	Bioflavonoids (mixed)	167.0	mg	38	Vanadium	23.0	ug
19	Phenolic compounds	8.0	mg	39	Zinc	6.0	mg
20	Procyanidolic Oligomers	23.0	mg		* Not Available in Canadian Products		

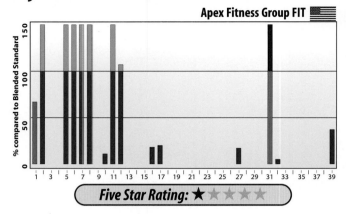

Apex Fitness Group FIT

Five Star Rating: ★ ☆ ☆ ☆ ☆

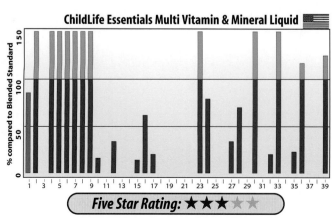

Axcan Pharma ADEKs Tablets

Five Star Rating: ★ ☆ ☆ ☆ ☆

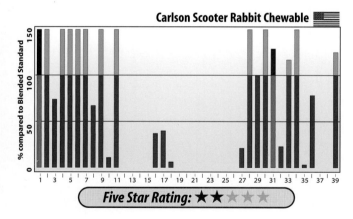

Body Wise Tiger Vites

Five Star Rating: ★ ★ ☆ ☆ ☆

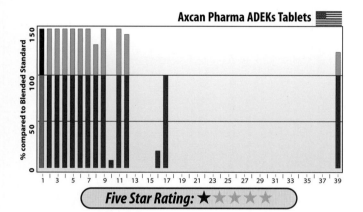

Carlson Scooter Rabbit Chewable

Five Star Rating: ★ ★ ☆ ☆ ☆

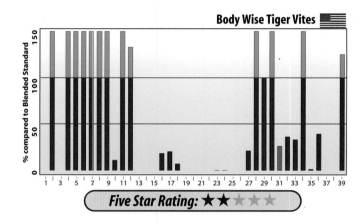

Centrum Junior Complete

Five Star Rating: ★ ☆ ☆ ☆ ☆

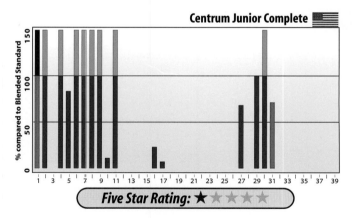

ChildLife Essentials Multi Vitamin & Mineral Liquid

Five Star Rating: ★ ★ ★ ☆ ☆

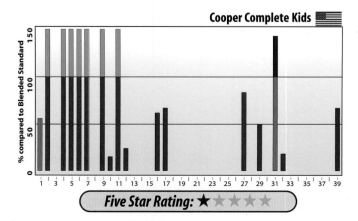

Cooper Complete Kids

Five Star Rating: ★ ☆ ☆ ☆ ☆

Graphical Comparisons to the Adjusted Blended Standard

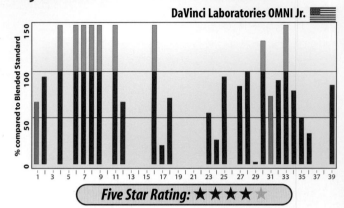

Country Life Dolphin Pals

Five Star Rating: ★ ★ ★ ☆ ☆

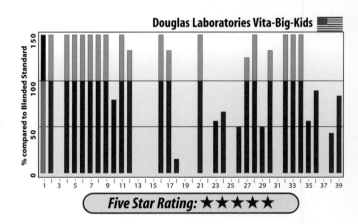

DaVinci Laboratories OMNI Jr.

Five Star Rating: ★ ★ ★ ★ ☆

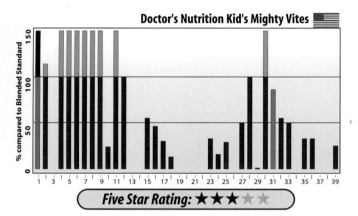

Doctor's Nutrition Kid's Mighty Vites

Five Star Rating: ★ ★ ★ ☆ ☆

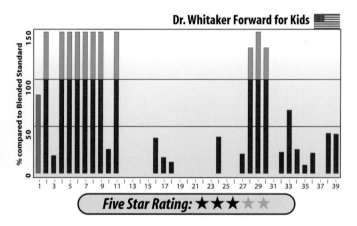

Douglas Laboratories Vita-Big-Kids

Five Star Rating: ★ ★ ★ ★ ★

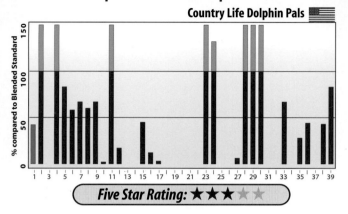

Dr. Whitaker Forward for Kids

Five Star Rating: ★ ★ ★ ☆ ☆

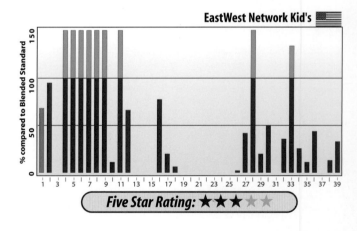

EastWest Network Kid's

Five Star Rating: ★ ★ ★ ☆ ☆

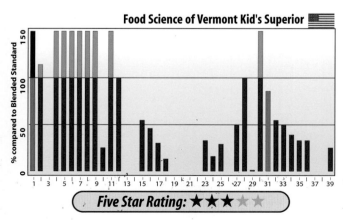

Food Science of Vermont Kid's Superior

Five Star Rating: ★ ★ ★ ☆ ☆

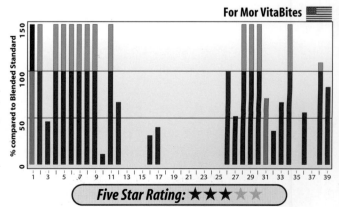

For Mor VitaBites

Five Star Rating: ★ ★ ★ ☆ ☆

Graphical Comparisons to the Adjusted Blended Standard

Adjusted Blended Standard

#	Nutrient	Amount	Unit	#	Nutrient	Amount	Unit
1	Vitamin A	1500.0	IU	21	n-Acetyl-l-Cysteine	17.0	mg
2	Vitamin D3	105.0	IU	22	l-Carnitine	225.0	mg
3	Vitamin K*	54.0	ug	23	Choline	18.0	mg
4	Biotin	12.0	ug	24	Inositol	38.0	mg
5	Folic Acid	120.0	ug	25	Lecithin	105.0	mg
6	Vitamin B$_1$	0.6	mg	26	Boron*	1.0	mg
7	Vitamin B$_2$	0.6	mg	27	Calcium	240.0	mg
8	Vitamin B$_3$ complex	7.5	mg	28	Chromium	15.0	ug
9	Vitamin B$_5$	3.0	mg	29	Copper	1.0	mg
10	Vitamin B$_6$	19.0	mg	30	Iodine	30.0	ug
11	Vitamin B$_{12}$	1.2	ug	31	Iron	7.0	mg
12	beta-Carotene	3750.0	IU	32	Magnesium	110.0	mg
13	Coenzyme Q$_{10}$	14.0	mg	33	Manganese	1.5	mg
14	Lipoic Acid	11.0	mg	34	Molybdenum	19.0	ug
15	Para-Aminobenzoic Acid	11.0	mg	35	Potassium	90.0	mg
16	Vitamin C	325.0	mg	36	Selenium	45.0	ug
17	Vitamin E	150.0	IU	37	Silicon	2.0	mg
18	Bioflavonoids (mixed)	167.0	mg	38	Vanadium	23.0	ug
19	Phenolic compounds	8.0	mg	39	Zinc	6.0	mg
20	Procyanidolic Oligomers	23.0	mg		* Not Available in Canadian Products		

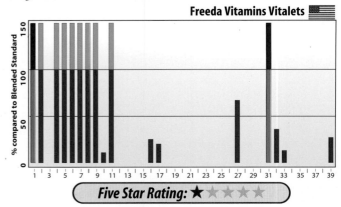

Freeda Vitamins Vitalets

Five Star Rating: ★ ☆ ☆ ☆ ☆

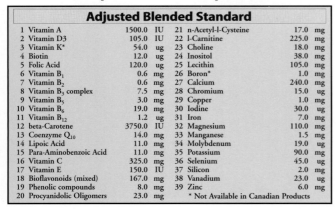

FreeLife DinoPals

Five Star Rating: ★ ★ ★ ☆ ☆

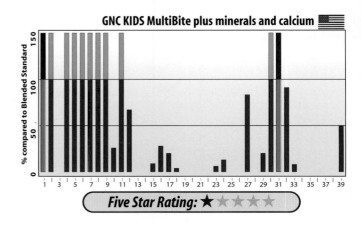

GNC KIDS MultiBite plus minerals and calcium

Five Star Rating: ★ ☆ ☆ ☆ ☆

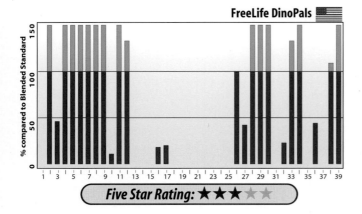

Goldshield Elite Herbal Supplements Kid's Stuff

Five Star Rating: ★ ☆ ☆ ☆ ☆

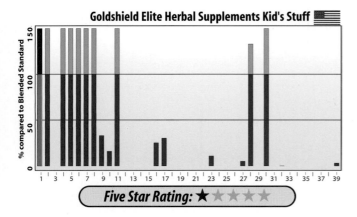

Great Earth Teddy Children's Chewables

Five Star Rating: ★ ★ ☆ ☆ ☆

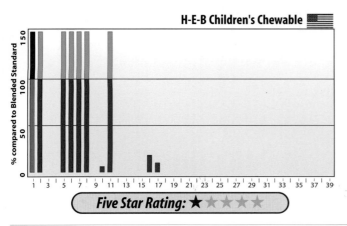

H-E-B Children's Chewable

Five Star Rating: ★ ☆ ☆ ☆ ☆

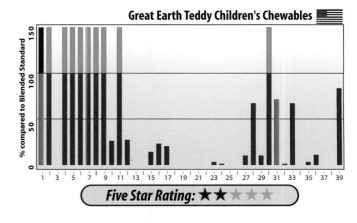

Herbalife Dinomins

Five Star Rating: ★ ★ ☆ ☆ ☆

Graphical Comparisons to the Adjusted Blended Standard

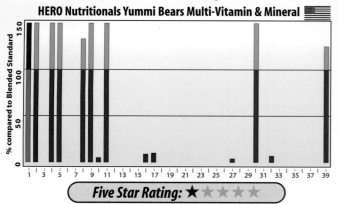

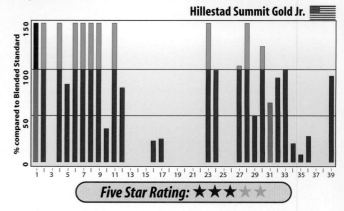

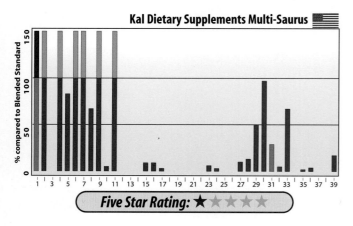

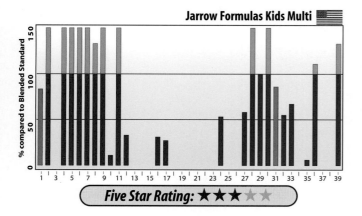

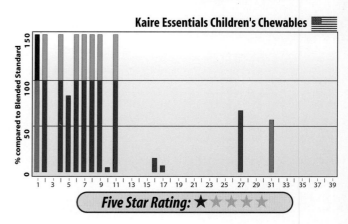

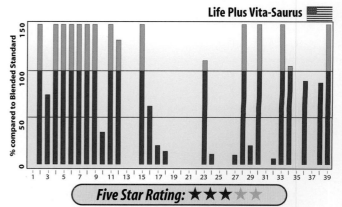

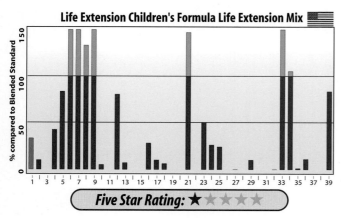

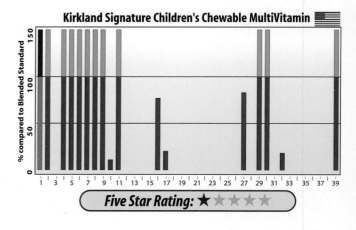

Graphical Comparisons to the Adjusted Blended Standard

Adjusted Blended Standard

1	Vitamin A	1500.0	IU	21	n-Acetyl-l-Cysteine	17.0	mg
2	Vitamin D3	105.0	IU	22	l-Carnitine	225.0	mg
3	Vitamin K*	54.0	ug	23	Choline	18.0	mg
4	Biotin	12.0	ug	24	Inositol	38.0	mg
5	Folic Acid	120.0	ug	25	Lecithin	105.0	mg
6	Vitamin B$_1$	0.6	mg	26	Boron*	1.0	mg
7	Vitamin B$_2$	0.6	mg	27	Calcium	240.0	mg
8	Vitamin B$_3$ complex	7.5	mg	28	Chromium	15.0	ug
9	Vitamin B$_5$	3.0	mg	29	Copper	1.0	mg
10	Vitamin B$_6$	19.0	mg	30	Iodine	30.0	ug
11	Vitamin B$_{12}$	1.2	ug	31	Iron	7.0	mg
12	beta-Carotene	3750.0	IU	32	Magnesium	110.0	mg
13	Coenzyme Q$_{10}$	14.0	mg	33	Manganese	1.5	mg
14	Lipoic Acid	11.0	mg	34	Molybdenum	19.0	ug
15	Para-Aminobenzoic Acid	11.0	mg	35	Potassium	90.0	mg
16	Vitamin C	325.0	mg	36	Selenium	45.0	ug
17	Vitamin E	150.0	IU	37	Silicon	2.0	mg
18	Bioflavonoids (mixed)	167.0	mg	38	Vanadium	23.0	ug
19	Phenolic compounds	8.0	mg	39	Zinc	6.0	mg
20	Procyanidolic Oligomers	23.0	mg		* Not Available in Canadian Products		

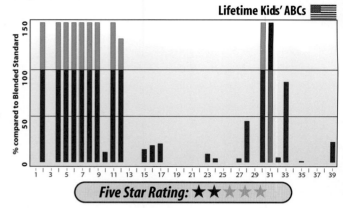

Lifetime Kids' ABCs

Five Star Rating: ★★☆☆☆

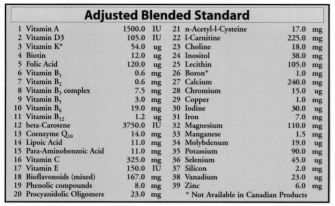

Maximum Living Little Angels

Five Star Rating: ★★☆☆☆

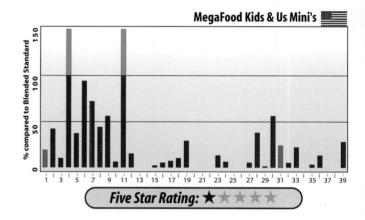

MegaFood Kids & Us Mini's

Five Star Rating: ★☆☆☆☆

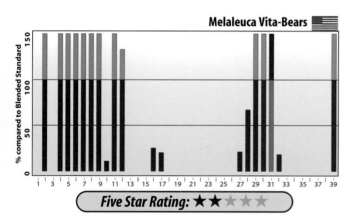

Melaleuca Vita-Bears

Five Star Rating: ★★☆☆☆

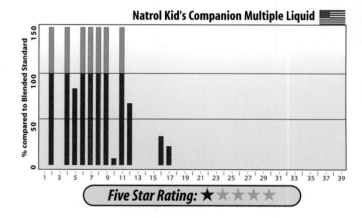

Natrol Kid's Companion Multiple Liquid

Five Star Rating: ★☆☆☆☆

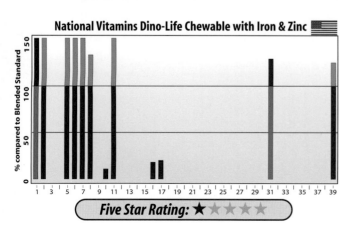

National Vitamins Dino-Life Chewable with Iron & Zinc

Five Star Rating: ★☆☆☆☆

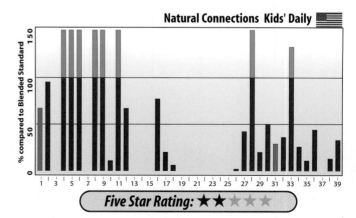

Natural Connections Kids' Daily

Five Star Rating: ★★☆☆☆

Graphical Comparisons to the Adjusted Blended Standard

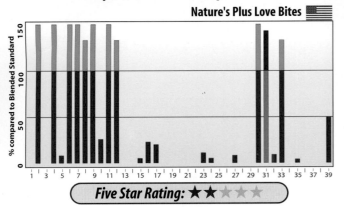

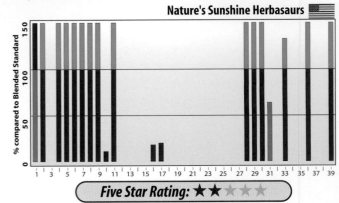

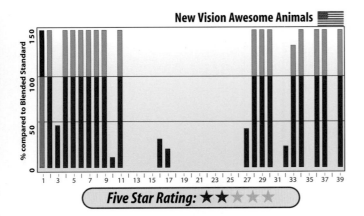

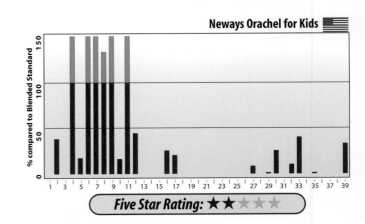

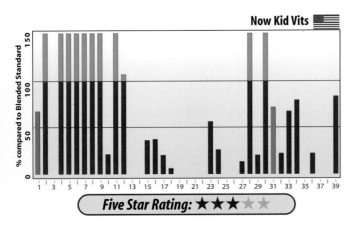

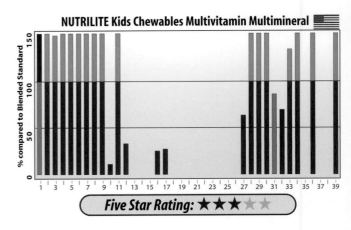

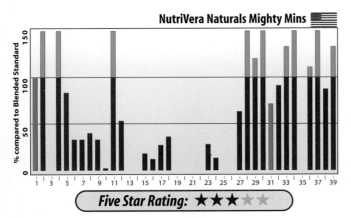

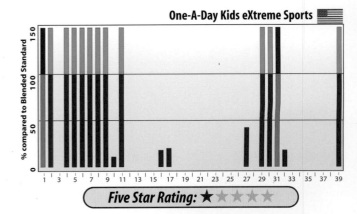

Graphical Comparisons to the Adjusted Blended Standard

Adjusted Blended Standard

1	Vitamin A	1500.0 IU	21	n-Acetyl-l-Cysteine	17.0 mg
2	Vitamin D3	105.0 IU	22	l-Carnitine	225.0 mg
3	Vitamin K*	54.0 ug	23	Choline	18.0 mg
4	Biotin	12.0 ug	24	Inositol	38.0 mg
5	Folic Acid	120.0 ug	25	Lecithin	105.0 mg
6	Vitamin B$_1$	0.6 mg	26	Boron*	1.0 mg
7	Vitamin B$_2$	0.6 mg	27	Calcium	240.0 mg
8	Vitamin B$_3$ complex	7.5 mg	28	Chromium	15.0 ug
9	Vitamin B$_5$	3.0 mg	29	Copper	1.0 mg
10	Vitamin B$_6$	19.0 mg	30	Iodine	30.0 mg
11	Vitamin B$_{12}$	1.2 mg	31	Iron	7.0 mg
12	beta-Carotene	3750.0 IU	32	Magnesium	110.0 mg
13	Coenzyme Q$_{10}$	14.0 mg	33	Manganese	1.5 mg
14	Lipoic Acid	11.0 mg	34	Molybdenum	19.0 ug
15	Para-Aminobenzoic Acid	11.0 mg	35	Potassium	90.0 mg
16	Vitamin C	325.0 mg	36	Selenium	45.0 ug
17	Vitamin E	150.0 IU	37	Silicon	2.0 mg
18	Bioflavonoids (mixed)	167.0 mg	38	Vanadium	23.0 ug
19	Phenolic compounds	8.0 mg	39	Zinc	6.0 mg
20	Procyanidolic Oligomers	23.0 mg		* Not Available in Canadian Products	

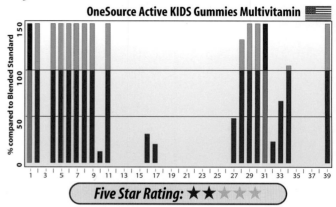

OneSource Active KIDS Gummies Multivitamin

Five Star Rating: ★★☆☆☆

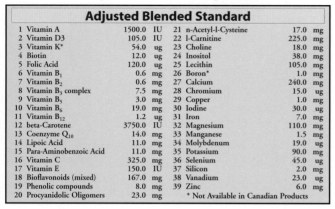

Pharmanex Jungamals

Five Star Rating: ★★★★☆

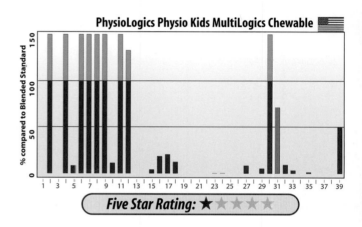

PhysioLogics Physio Kids MultiLogics Chewable

Five Star Rating: ★☆☆☆☆

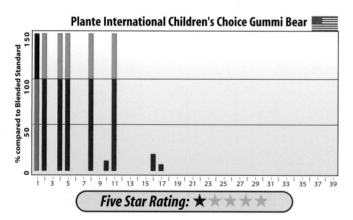

Plante International Children's Choice Gummi Bear

Five Star Rating: ★☆☆☆☆

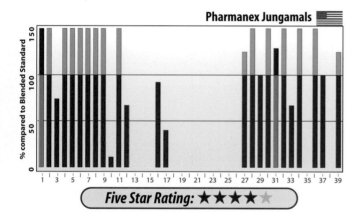

Priority One School Days-Priority Vegetarian Tab

Five Star Rating: ★★☆☆☆

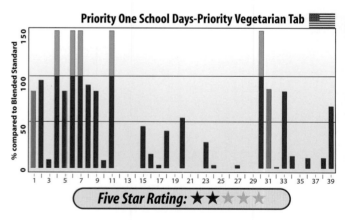

ProThera VitaTab Chewable

Five Star Rating: ★★★★☆

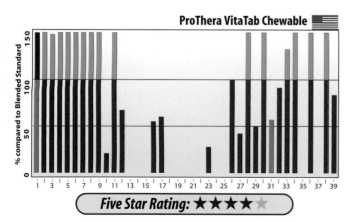

Puritan's Pride Animal Chews

Five Star Rating: ★★☆☆☆

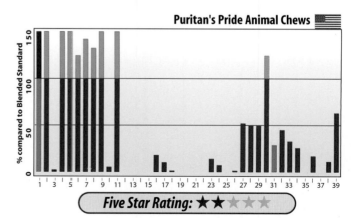

Graphical Comparisons to the Adjusted Blended Standard

Rainbow Light Kids' One MultiStars

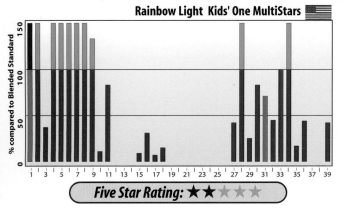

Five Star Rating: ★★☆☆☆

Rite Aid Children's Chewable Vitamins Complete

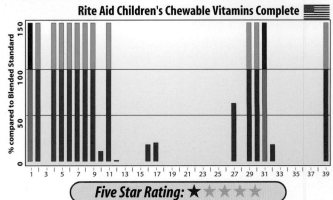

Five Star Rating: ★☆☆☆☆

Rx Vitamins Children's Multi-Vitamins

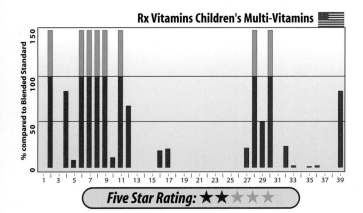

Five Star Rating: ★★☆☆☆

Schiff Children's Chewable

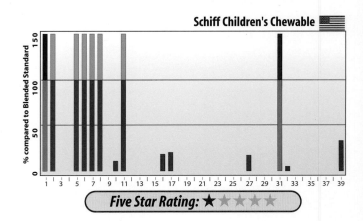

Five Star Rating: ★☆☆☆☆

Sesame Street Complete

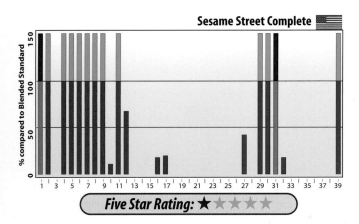

Five Star Rating: ★☆☆☆☆

Shaklee Vita-Lea for Children

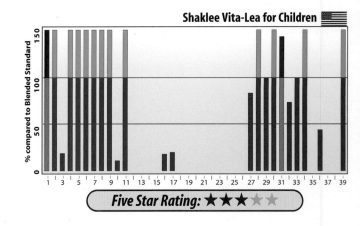

Five Star Rating: ★★★☆☆

Sisu Mini-Vits

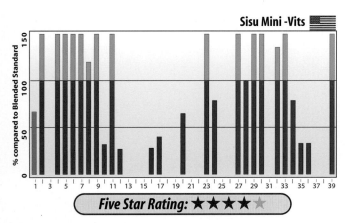

Five Star Rating: ★★★★☆

Solaray Children's Chewable

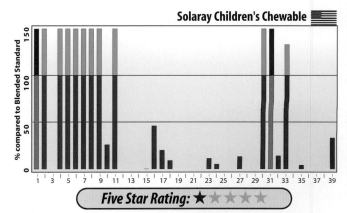

Five Star Rating: ★☆☆☆☆

Graphical Comparisons to the Adjusted Blended Standard

Adjusted Blended Standard

1	Vitamin A	1500.0	IU	21	n-Acetyl-l-Cysteine	17.0	mg
2	Vitamin D3	105.0	IU	22	l-Carnitine	225.0	mg
3	Vitamin K*	54.0	ug	23	Choline	18.0	mg
4	Biotin	12.0	ug	24	Inositol	38.0	mg
5	Folic Acid	120.0	ug	25	Lecithin	105.0	mg
6	Vitamin B$_1$	0.6	mg	26	Boron*	1.0	mg
7	Vitamin B$_2$	0.6	mg	27	Calcium	240.0	mg
8	Vitamin B$_3$ complex	7.5	mg	28	Chromium	15.0	ug
9	Vitamin B$_5$	3.0	mg	29	Copper	1.0	mg
10	Vitamin B$_6$	19.0	mg	30	Iodine	30.0	ug
11	Vitamin B$_{12}$	1.2	ug	31	Iron	7.0	mg
12	beta-Carotene	3750.0	IU	32	Magnesium	110.0	mg
13	Coenzyme Q$_{10}$	14.0	mg	33	Manganese	1.5	mg
14	Lipoic Acid	11.0	mg	34	Molybdenum	19.0	ug
15	Para-Aminobenzoic Acid	11.0	mg	35	Potassium	90.0	mg
16	Vitamin C	325.0	mg	36	Selenium	45.0	ug
17	Vitamin E	150.0	IU	37	Silicon	2.0	mg
18	Bioflavonoids (mixed)	167.0	mg	38	Vanadium	23.0	ug
19	Phenolic compounds	8.0	mg	39	Zinc	6.0	mg
20	Procyanidolic Oligomers	23.0	mg		* Not Available in Canadian Products		

Solgar Kangavites
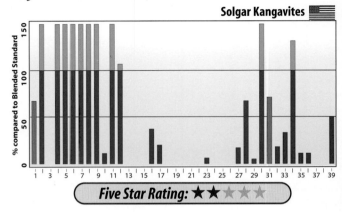

Five Star Rating: ★★☆☆☆

Source Naturals Mega-Kid Multiple
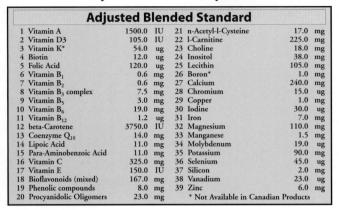

Five Star Rating: ★★★★☆

Sundown Kids Super Heroes
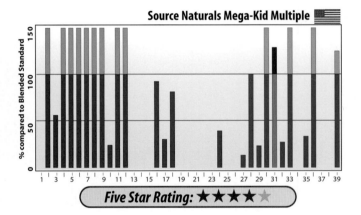

Five Star Rating: ★☆☆☆☆

SuperNutrition Perfect Kids
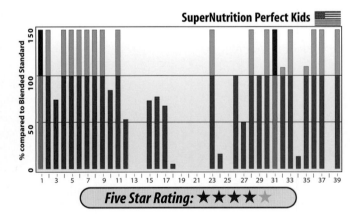

Five Star Rating: ★★★★☆

SupraLife Kid's Toddy
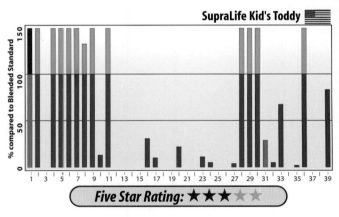

Five Star Rating: ★★★☆☆

Symmetry Future Star
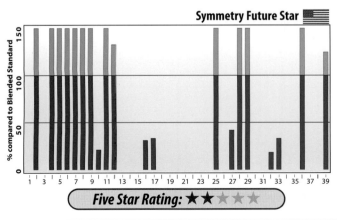

Five Star Rating: ★★☆☆☆

T.J. Clark Children's Complete Vitamino Advanced Formula
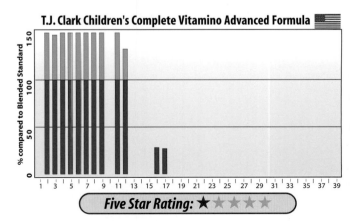

Five Star Rating: ★☆☆☆☆

Graphical Comparisons to the Adjusted Blended Standard

Thompson Children's Chewable Multivitamin

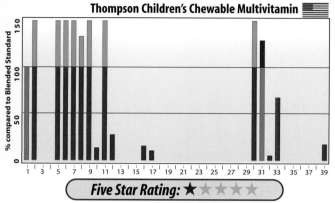

Five Star Rating: ★ ☆ ☆ ☆ ☆

Thorne Research Children's Basic Nutrients with Copper & Iron

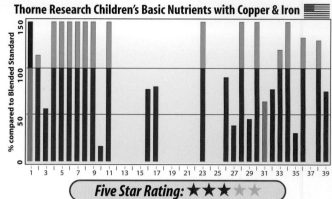

Five Star Rating: ★ ★ ★ ☆ ☆

Trace Minerals Research Liquimins Kids Multi

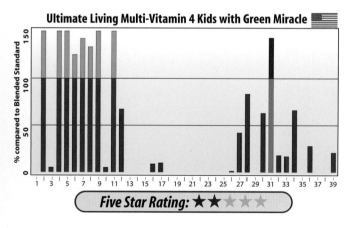

Five Star Rating: ★ ☆ ☆ ☆ ☆

Ultimate Health Children's Chewables

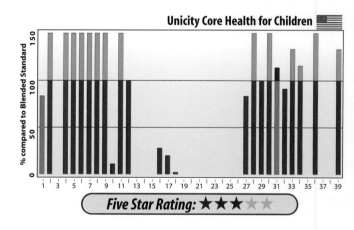

Five Star Rating: ★ ★ ☆ ☆ ☆

Ultimate Living Multi-Vitamin 4 Kids with Green Miracle

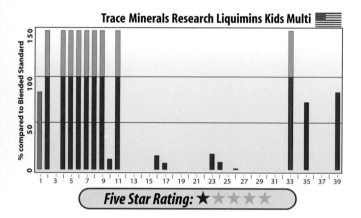

Five Star Rating: ★ ★ ☆ ☆ ☆

Unicity Core Health for Children

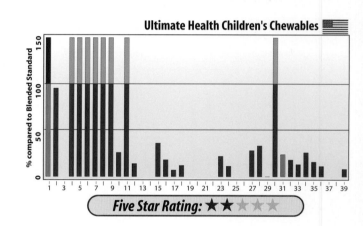

Five Star Rating: ★ ★ ★ ☆ ☆

USANA Health Sciences Usanimals

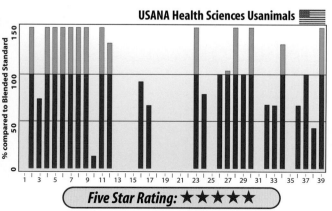

Five Star Rating: ★ ★ ★ ★ ★

Växa Buddies

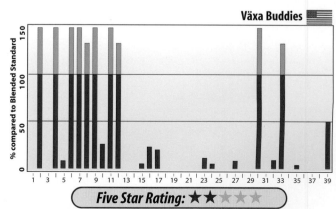

Five Star Rating: ★ ★ ☆ ☆ ☆

Graphical Comparisons to the Adjusted Blended Standard

Adjusted Blended Standard

1	Vitamin A	1500.0	IU	21	n-Acetyl-l-Cysteine	17.0	mg
2	Vitamin D3	105.0	IU	22	l-Carnitine	225.0	mg
3	Vitamin K*	54.0	ug	23	Choline	18.0	mg
4	Biotin	12.0	ug	24	Inositol	38.0	mg
5	Folic Acid	120.0	ug	25	Lecithin	105.0	mg
6	Vitamin B$_1$	0.6	mg	26	Boron*	1.0	mg
7	Vitamin B$_2$	0.6	mg	27	Calcium	240.0	mg
8	Vitamin B$_3$ complex	7.5	mg	28	Chromium	15.0	ug
9	Vitamin B$_5$	3.0	mg	29	Copper	1.0	mg
10	Vitamin B$_6$	19.0	mg	30	Iodine	30.0	ug
11	Vitamin B$_{12}$	1.2	ug	31	Iron	7.0	mg
12	beta-Carotene	3750.0	IU	32	Magnesium	110.0	mg
13	Coenzyme Q$_{10}$	14.0	mg	33	Manganese	1.5	mg
14	Lipoic Acid	11.0	mg	34	Molybdenum	19.0	ug
15	Para-Aminobenzoic Acid	11.0	mg	35	Potassium	90.0	mg
16	Vitamin C	325.0	mg	36	Selenium	45.0	ug
17	Vitamin E	150.0	IU	37	Silicon	2.0	mg
18	Bioflavonoids (mixed)	167.0	mg	38	Vanadium	23.0	ug
19	Phenolic compounds	8.0	mg	39	Zinc	6.0	mg
20	Procyanidolic Oligomers	23.0	mg		* Not Available in Canadian Products		

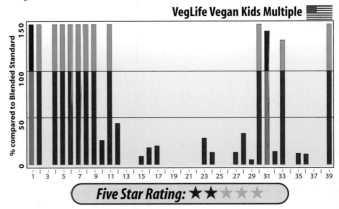

VegLife Vegan Kids Multiple

Five Star Rating: ★★☆☆☆

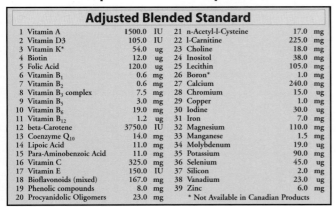

Vitamin Power Children's Multi-Vites with Minerals

Five Star Rating: ★☆☆☆☆

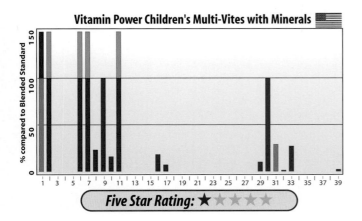

Vitamin Research Products Kids Essentials

Five Star Rating: ★★★★☆

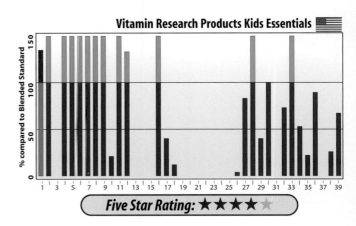

Vitamin Shoppe Vita-Bear Multiple

Five Star Rating: ★★☆☆☆

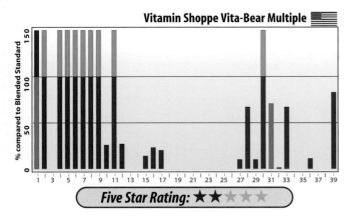

Vitamin World Children's Chewable Animal Chews

Five Star Rating: ★★☆☆☆

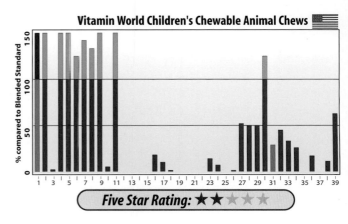

VitaminLab Children's Chewable

Five Star Rating: ★☆☆☆☆

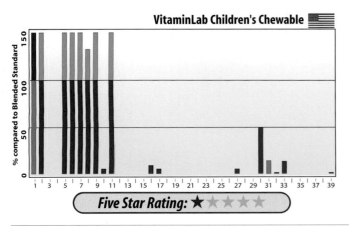

VitaMist Spray Vitamins Children's Multiple

Five Star Rating: ★☆☆☆☆

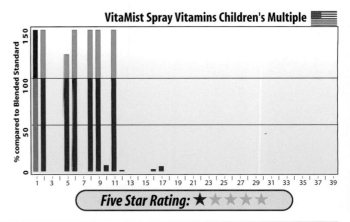

Graphical Comparisons to the Adjusted Blended Standard

Viva Life Science Viva EZ Kids

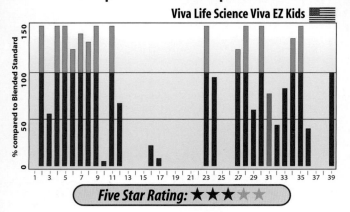

Five Star Rating: ★★★☆☆

Watkins Children's Chewable

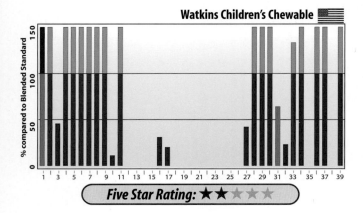

Five Star Rating: ★★☆☆☆

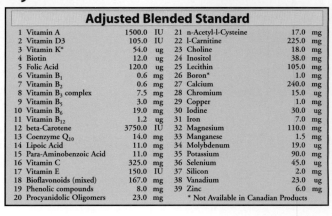

Adjusted Blended Standard

#				#			
1	Vitamin A	1500.0	IU	21	n-Acetyl-l-Cysteine	17.0	mg
2	Vitamin D3	105.0	IU	22	l-Carnitine	225.0	mg
3	Vitamin K*	54.0	ug	23	Choline	18.0	mg
4	Biotin	12.0	ug	24	Inositol	38.0	mg
5	Folic Acid	120.0	ug	25	Lecithin	105.0	mg
6	Vitamin B$_1$	0.6	mg	26	Boron*	1.0	mg
7	Vitamin B$_2$	0.6	mg	27	Calcium	240.0	mg
8	Vitamin B$_3$ complex	7.5	mg	28	Chromium	15.0	ug
9	Vitamin B$_5$	3.0	mg	29	Copper	1.0	mg
10	Vitamin B$_6$	19.0	mg	30	Iodine	30.0	ug
11	Vitamin B$_{12}$	1.2	ug	31	Iron	7.0	mg
12	beta-Carotene	3750.0	IU	32	Magnesium	110.0	mg
13	Coenzyme Q$_{10}$	14.0	mg	33	Manganese	1.5	mg
14	Lipoic Acid	11.0	mg	34	Molybdenum	19.0	ug
15	Para-Aminobenzoic Acid	11.0	mg	35	Potassium	90.0	mg
16	Vitamin C	325.0	mg	36	Selenium	45.0	ug
17	Vitamin E	150.0	IU	37	Silicon	2.0	mg
18	Bioflavonoids (mixed)	167.0	mg	38	Vanadium	23.0	ug
19	Phenolic compounds	8.0	mg	39	Zinc	6.0	mg
20	Procyanidolic Oligomers	23.0	mg		* Not Available in Canadian Products		

Appendices

- Alphabetical listing of products reviewed
- Product-score listing of products reviewed

Appendix A: Products sorted by Company Name

Company Name CANADA	Product Name CANADA	Raw Score (out of 14) CANADA	Percent Score CANADA	Dosages & Considerations
Bayer	Bugs Bunny and Friends Complete	2.3	16	
Bayer	Flintstones Multiple Vitamins Complete with Calcium & Iron	2.3	16	
Carter-Horner Corp.	Infantol	2.1	15	
Centrum	Junior Complete	2.5	18	
Club Vitamin	Best	5.3	38	
Equate	Complete	2.3	16	DOSAGE DERIVED
Essaim	Multivitamins Children's Chewable	1.7	12	
Essaim	Multivitamines à Croquer pour Enfants	2.3	16	
Flora/Salus	Kindervital Multivitamin for Children	2.2	15	
GNC Kids	Mega Kids	2.8	20	
GNC Kids	Children's Multiple Vitamins Plus Minerals	3.4	24	
Goldshield Elite Herbal Supplements	Kid's Stuff	2.9	21	
Jamieson	Arthur	3.0	21	
Jamieson	Arthur Iron Fortified Formula	3.3	24	
Kaire Essentials	Children's Chewables	2.2	16	
Kal Dietary Supplements	StegoVites	3.4	24	
Kid Bear	Vegetarian Multi-Vitamin & Mineral	2.6	19	
Kirkland Signature	Children's Chewable MultiVitamin	2.8	20	
Kirkland Signature	Multivitamins for Children	2.3	16	
Life	for Kids Only	2.2	16	
Lifestyles	Lifecycles Children's Chewables	5.4	39	
Li'l Critters	Gummy Vites	2.6	18	
London Drugs	Children's Chewable Multi Vitamins Regular	1.6	12	
Mr. Tumee	Gelatin Free Multi-Vitamin Supplement Gumee	3.1	22	
Natural Factors	Big Friends	8.2	58	
Natural Factors	Learning Factors Daily Nutrient Boost	8.1	58	
Natural Source	Kids Chewable	2.8	20	
Now	Kid Vits	7.2	52	
Nu-Life	NuBears	6.5	47	
Nutrilite	Kids Chewable Multivitamin/Iron Supplement	3.2	23	
Nutrition Now	Rhino Chewy Vites	2.1	15	
Personnelle	Multivitamines à Croquer Enfants Formule Complète	2.3	16	DOSAGE DERIVED
Plante International	Children's Choice Gummi Bear	2.3	16	
Quest	Kids	5.2	37	
Safeway Select	Children's Chewable Vitamins Complete with Calcium & Iron	2.3	16	
SISU	Mini -Vits	9.8	70	
Solaray	Children's Chewable	3.8	27	
Sunkist Vitamins	Sunkids	2.8	20	
Swiss Natural Sources	Children's Choice Iron Free	4.9	35	
Trophic	Chewable Multi Vitamin	3.4	24	
Trophic	Chewable Multi Vitamin with Iron	2.6	19	
Truly Health	Children's Chewable Multi-vitamins with Iron	1.7	12	
USANA Health Sciences	Usanimals	10.8	77	
Watkins	Watkins Jr.	4.9	35	
Western Family	Children's Chewable	2.8	20	
USA	**USA**	**USA**	**USA**	
21st Century	Zoo Friends with Extra C	2.7	19	
21st Century	Zoo Friends	2.6	19	
21st Century	Zoo Friends with Iron	2.6	19	
21st Century	Zoo Friends Complete	2.8	20	
4Life	TF Kids	7.1	51	
Allergy Research Group	Children's Multi-Vi-Min	6.5	46	BASED ON 50 LBS.
American Health	Chewy Bears and Friends	4.9	35	
AMNI	Kids	6.8	48	
Anabolic Laboratories	Aved-Eze	7.6	54	
Andrew Lessman	Children's Complete Vitamin and Mineral Drink	6.8	49	
Apex Fitness Group	Fit	3.6	26	
Axcan Pharma	Adeks Tablets	2.5	18	
Body Wise	Tiger Vites	5.8	41	
Carlson	Scooter Rabbit Chewable	5.6	40	
Centrum	Junior Complete	2.5	18	
ChildLife Essentials	Multi Vitamin & Mineral Liquid	7.1	51	
Cooper Complete	Kids	3.9	28	
Country Life	Dolphin Pals	6.3	45	
Country Life	Tall Tree Children's Chewable	4.5	32	
DaVinci Laboratories	Kid's Mighty Vites	7.0	50	
DaVinci Laboratories	Omni Jr.	8.5	61	
Doctor's Nutrition	Kid's Mighty Vites	7.0	50	
Douglas Laboratories	Astra-Vites	2.8	20	
Douglas Laboratories	Basic Preventive Junior	9.8	70	
Douglas Laboratories	Children's Essentials	9.4	67	
Douglas Laboratories	Vita-Big-Kids	11.4	81	

Douglas Laboratories	Vita-Kids	6.8	48	
Dr. Whitaker	Forward for Kids	6.3	45	
EastWest Network	Kid's	6.8	48	
Food Science of Vermont	Kid's Superior	7.0	50	
For Mor	VitaBites	6.8	49	
Freeda Vitamins	Vitalets	3.6	26	
FreeLife	DinoPals	6.7	48	
GNC Kids	MultiBite Plus Minerals and Calcium	3.8	27	
Goldshield Elite Herbal Supplements	Kid's Stuff	2.9	21	
Great Earth	Teddy Children's Chewables	4.5	32	
H-E-B	Children's Chewable	2.6	19	
Herbalife	Dinomins	4.2	30	
Hero Nutritionals	Yummi Bears Multi-Vitamin & Mineral	3.1	22	
Hero Nutritionals	Yummi Sourz	2.6	19	
Hero Nutritionals	Yummi Bears Vegetarian Multi-Vitamin & Mineral	3.1	22	
Hillestad	CC's Children's Chewables	3.2	23	
Hillestad	Summit Gold Jr.	7.7	55	
Jarrow Formulas	Kids Multi	7.4	53	
Kaire Essentials	Children's Chewables	2.2	16	
Kal Dietary Supplements	Multi-Saurus	3.2	23	
Kirkland Signature	Children's Chewable MultiVitamin	2.8	20	
Life Extension	Children's Formula Life Extension Mix	3.4	24	
Life Plus	Vita-Saurus	7.4	53	
LifeTime	Kids' ABCs	4.3	31	
Maximum Living	Little Angels	5.5	40	
MegaFood	Kids & Us Mini's	3.4	24	
Melaleuca	Vita-Bears	4.6	33	
National Vitamins	Dino-Life Chewable Multi-Vitamins with Extra C	2.4	17	
National Vitamins	Dino-Life Chewable Multi-Vitamins with Iron & Zinc	2.4	17	
Natrol	Kid's Companion Multiple Liquid	2.9	21	
Natural Connections	Kids' Daily	5.9	42	
Nature's Plus	Animal Parade Gummies	3.4	24	
Nature's Plus	Children's Vita-Gels	3.4	24	
Nature's Plus	Love Bites	4.3	31	
Nature's Sunshine	Herbasaurs	5.2	37	
New Vision	Awesome Animals	5.7	41	
Neways	Orachel for Kids	4.4	31	
Now	Kid Vits	6.8	49	
Nutrilite	Kids Chewables Multivitamin Multimineral	6.4	46	
NutriVera Naturals	Mighty Mins	7.1	51	
One-A-Day Kids	Bugs Bunny and Friends Complete	2.8	20	
One-A-Day Kids	Extreme Sports	3.3	24	
One-A-Day Kids	Fizzy Vites	3.4	24	
OneSource	Active Kids Gummies Multivitamin	4.1	29	
Pharmanex	Jungamals	9.4	67	
PhysioLogics	Physio Kids MultiLogics Chewable	3.6	26	
Plante International	Children's Choice Gummi Bear	2.3	16	
Priority One Nutritional Supplements	School Days-Priority Vegetarian Tab	4.3	31	
ProThera	VitaTab Chewable	9.7	69	
Puritan's Pride	Animal Chews	4.9	35	
Rainbow Light	Kids' One MultiStars	5.8	42	
Rite Aid	Children's Chewable Vitamins Complete	2.8	20	
Rx Vitamins	Children's Multi-Vitamins	4.1	29	
Schiff	Children's Chewable	2.9	20	
Schiff	Children's Multivitamin Liquid	2.7	20	
Sesame Street	Complete	3.5	25	
Shaklee	Vita-Lea for Children	6.5	46	
Shaklee	Vita-Lea Ocean Wonders	5.9	42	
SISU	Mini -Vits	8.2	59	
Solaray	Children's Chewable	3.8	27	
Solgar	Kangavites	5.1	36	
Source Naturals	Mega-Kid Multiple	9.1	65	
Sundown Kids	Complete	2.5	18	
Sundown Kids	Super Heroes	3.5	25	
Super Nutrition	Perfect Kids	9.6	69	
SupraLife	Kid's Toddy	6.5	46	
Symmetry	Future Star	5.4	39	
T.J. Clark	Children's Complete Vitamino Advanced Formula	3.7	26	
Thompson	Children's Chewable Multivitamin	3.6	26	
Thorne Research	Childrens' Basic Nutrients with Copper & Iron	7.6	54	
Trace Minerals Research	Liquimins Kids Multi	3.4	24	
Ultimate Health	Children's Chewables	4.6	33	
Ultimate Living	Multi-Vitamin 4 Kids with Green Miracle	4.3	30	
Unicity	Core Health for Children	7.1	51	
USANA Health Sciences	Usanimals	10.6	76	
Växa	Buddies	4.2	30	
VegLife	Vegan Kids Multiple	4.4	32	
Vitamin Power	Children's Multi-Vites with Minerals	2.1	15	DOSAGE DERIVED
Vitamin Research Products	Kids Essentials	8.5	60	
Vitamin Shoppe	Chewy Vita-Bear Multiple	2.7	19	

Vitamin Shoppe	Vita-Bear Multiple	4.5	32	
Vitamin World	Children's Chewable Animal Chews	4.9	35	
VitaminLab	Children's Chewable	2.6	19	
VitaMist Spray Vitamins	Children's Multiple	2.6	19	
Viva Life Science	Viva EZ Kids	7.1	51	
Viva Life Science	Viva Kids Plus	5.1	36	
Watkins	Children's Chewable	5.3	38	

Appendix B: Products sorted by Final Product Score

Company Name	Product Name	Raw Score (out of 14)	Percent Score	Dosages & Considerations
CANADA	**CANADA**	**CANADA**	**CANADA**	
USANA Health Sciences	Usanimals	10.8	77	
SISU	Mini -Vits	9.8	70	
Natural Factors	Big Friends	8.2	58	
Natural Factors	Learning Factors Daily Nutrient Boost	8.1	58	
Now	Kid Vits	7.2	52	
Nu-Life	NuBears	6.5	47	
Lifestyles	Lifecycles Children's Chewables	5.4	39	
Club Vitamin	Best	5.3	38	
Quest	Kids	5.2	37	
Swiss Natural Sources	Children's Choice Iron Free	4.9	35	
Watkins	Watkins Jr.	4.9	35	
Solaray	Children's Chewable	3.8	27	
GNC Kids	Children's Multiple Vitamins Plus Minerals	3.4	24	
Kal Dietary Supplements	StegoVites	3.4	24	
Trophic	Chewable Multi Vitamin	3.4	24	
Jamieson	Arthur Iron Fortified Formula	3.3	24	
Nutrilite	Kids Chewable Multivitamin/Iron Supplement	3.2	23	
Mr. Tumee	Gelatin Free Multi-Vitamin Supplement Gumee	3.1	22	
Jamieson	Arthur	3.0	21	
Goldshield Elite Herbal Supplements	Kid's Stuff	2.9	21	
Kirkland Signature	Children's Chewable MultiVitamin	2.8	20	
GNC Kids	Mega Kids	2.8	20	
Natural Source	Kids Chewable	2.8	20	
Sunkist Vitamins	Sunkids	2.8	20	
Western Family	Children's Chewable	2.8	20	
Kid Bear	Vegetarian Multi-Vitamin & Mineral	2.6	19	
Trophic	Chewable Multi Vitamin with Iron	2.6	19	
Li'l Critters	Gummy Vites	2.6	18	
Centrum	Junior Complete	2.5	18	
Bayer	Bugs Bunny and Friends Complete	2.3	16	
Bayer	Flintstones Multiple Vitamins Complete with Calcium & Iron	2.3	16	
Equate	Complete	2.3	16	DOSAGE DERIVED
Essaim	Multivitamines à Croquer pour Enfants	2.3	16	
Kirkland Signature	Multivitamins for Children	2.3	16	
Personnelle	Multivitamines à Croquer Enfants Formule Complète	2.3	16	DOSAGE DERIVED
Plante International	Children's Choice Gummi Bear	2.3	16	
Safeway Select	Children's Chewable Vitamins Complete with Calcium & Iron	2.3	16	
Kaire Essentials	Children's Chewables	2.2	16	
Life	for Kids Only	2.2	16	
Flora/Salus	Kindervital Multivitamin for Children	2.2	15	
Nutrition Now	Rhino Chewy Vites	2.1	15	
Carter-Horner Corp.	Infantol	2.1	15	
Essaim	Multivitamins Children's Chewable	1.7	12	
Truly Health	Children's Chewable Multi-vitamins with Iron	1.7	12	
London Drugs	Children's Chewable Multi Vitamins Regular	1.6	12	
USA	**USA**	**USA**	**USA**	
Douglas Laboratories	Vita-Big-Kids	11.4	81	
USANA Health Sciences	Usanimals	10.6	76	
Douglas Laboratories	Basic Preventive Junior	9.8	70	
ProThera	VitaTab Chewable	9.7	69	
Super Nutrition	Perfect Kids	9.6	69	
Douglas Laboratories	Children's Essentials	9.4	67	
Pharmanex	Jungamals	9.4	67	
Source Naturals	Mega-Kid Multiple	9.1	65	
DaVinci Laboratories	Omni Jr.	8.5	61	
Vitamin Research Products	Kids Essentials	8.5	60	
SISU	Mini -Vits	8.2	59	
Hillestad	Summit Gold Jr.	7.7	55	
Anabolic Laboratories	Aved-Eze	7.6	54	
Thorne Research	Childrens' Basic Nutrients with Copper & Iron	7.6	54	
Life Plus	Vita-Saurus	7.4	53	
Jarrow Formulas	Kids Multi	7.4	53	
4Life	TF Kids	7.1	51	
Unicity	Core Health for Children	7.1	51	
ChildLife Essentials	Multi Vitamin & Mineral Liquid	7.1	51	
NutriVera Naturals	Mighty Mins	7.1	51	
Viva Life Science	Viva EZ Kids	7.1	51	
DaVinci Laboratories	Kid's Mighty Vites	7.0	50	
Food Science of Vermont	Kid's Superior	7.0	50	
Doctor's Nutrition	Kid's Mighty Vites	7.0	50	
For Mor	VitaBites	6.8	49	
Now	Kid Vits	6.8	49	
Andrew Lessman	Children's Complete Vitamin and Mineral Drink	6.8	49	

AMNI	**Kids**	6.8	48	
Douglas Laboratories	**Vita-Kids**	6.8	48	
EastWest Network	**Kid's**	6.8	48	
FreeLife	**DinoPals**	6.7	48	
Allergy Research Group	**Children's Multi-Vi-Min**	6.5	46	**BASED ON 50 LBS.**
Shaklee	**Vita-Lea for Children**	6.5	46	
SupraLife	**Kid's Toddy**	6.5	46	
Nutrilite	**Kids Chewables Multivitamin Multimineral**	6.4	46	
Dr. Whitaker	**Forward for Kids**	6.3	45	
Country Life	**Dolphin Pals**	6.3	45	
Natural Connections	**Kids' Daily**	5.9	42	
Shaklee	**Vita-Lea Ocean Wonders**	5.9	42	
Rainbow Light	**Kids' One MultiStars**	5.8	42	
Body Wise	**Tiger Vites**	5.8	41	
New Vision	**Awesome Animals**	5.7	41	
Carlson	**Scooter Rabbit Chewable**	5.6	40	
Maximum Living	**Little Angels**	5.5	40	
Symmetry	**Future Star**	5.4	39	
Watkins	**Children's Chewable**	5.3	38	
Nature's Sunshine	**Herbasaurs**	5.2	37	
Viva Life Science	**Viva Kids Plus**	5.1	36	
Solgar	**Kangavites**	5.1	36	
American Health	**Chewy Bears and Friends**	4.9	35	
Puritan's Pride	**Animal Chews**	4.9	35	
Vitamin World	**Children's Chewable Animal Chews**	4.9	35	
Ultimate Health	**Children's Chewables**	4.6	33	
Melaleuca	**Vita-Bears**	4.6	33	
Country Life	**Tall Tree Children's Chewable**	4.5	32	
Vitamin Shoppe	**Vita-Bear Multiple**	4.5	32	
Great Earth	**Teddy Children's Chewables**	4.5	32	
VegLife	**Vegan Kids Multiple**	4.4	32	
Neways	**Orachel for Kids**	4.4	31	
Priority One Nutritional Supplements	**School Days-Priority Vegetarian Tab**	4.3	31	
LifeTime	**Kids' ABCs**	4.3	31	
Nature's Plus	**Love Bites**	4.3	31	
Ultimate Living	**Multi-Vitamin 4 Kids with Green Miracle**	4.3	30	
Växa	**Buddies**	4.2	30	
Herbalife	**Dinomins**	4.2	30	
Rx Vitamins	**Children's Multi-Vitamins**	4.1	29	
OneSource	**Active Kids Gummies Multivitamin**	4.1	29	
Cooper Complete	**Kids**	3.9	28	
GNC Kids	**MultiBite Plus Minerals and Calcium**	3.8	27	
Solaray	**Children's Chewable**	3.8	27	
T.J. Clark	**Children's Complete Vitamino Advanced Formula**	3.7	26	
Thompson	**Children's Chewable Multivitamin**	3.6	26	
Freeda Vitamins	**Vitalets**	3.6	26	
Apex Fitness Group	**Fit**	3.6	26	
PhysioLogics	**Physio Kids MultiLogics Chewable**	3.6	26	
Sesame Street	**Complete**	3.5	25	
Sundown Kids	**Super Heroes**	3.5	25	
Trace Minerals Research	**Liquimins Kids Multi**	3.4	24	
Nature's Plus	**Animal Parade Gummies**	3.4	24	
Life Extension	**Children's Formula Life Extension Mix**	3.4	24	
MegaFood	**Kids & Us Mini's**	3.4	24	
Nature's Plus	**Children's Vita-Gels**	3.4	24	
One-A-Day Kids	**Fizzy Vites**	3.4	24	
One-A-Day Kids	**Extreme Sports**	3.3	24	
Hillestad	**CC's Children's Chewables**	3.2	23	
Kal Dietary Supplements	**Multi-Saurus**	3.2	23	
Hero Nutritionals	**Yummi Bears Multi-Vitamin & Mineral**	3.1	22	
Hero Nutritionals	**Yummi Bears Vegetarian Multi-Vitamin & Mineral**	3.1	22	
Goldshield Elite Herbal Supplements	**Kid's Stuff**	2.9	21	
Natrol	**Kid's Companion Multiple Liquid**	2.9	21	
Schiff	**Children's Chewable**	2.9	20	
Kirkland Signature	**Children's Chewable MultiVitamin**	2.8	20	
One-A-Day Kids	**Bugs Bunny and Friends Complete**	2.8	20	
Rite Aid	**Children's Chewable Vitamins Complete**	2.8	20	
21st Century	**Zoo Friends Complete**	2.8	20	
Douglas Laboratories	**Astra-Vites**	2.8	20	
Schiff	**Children's Multivitamin Liquid**	2.7	20	
Vitamin Shoppe	**Chewy Vita-Bear Multiple**	2.7	19	
21st Century	**Zoo Friends with Extra C**	2.7	19	
Hero Nutritionals	**Yummi Sourz**	2.6	19	
21st Century	**Zoo Friends**	2.6	19	
21st Century	**Zoo Friends with Iron**	2.6	19	
VitaminLab	**Children's Chewable**	2.6	19	
H-E-B	**Children's Chewable**	2.6	19	
VitaMist Spray Vitamins	**Children's Multiple**	2.6	19	
Sundown Kids	**Complete**	2.5	18	
Centrum	**Junior Complete**	2.5	18	

Axcan Pharma	Adeks Tablets	2.5	18	
National Vitamins	Dino-Life Chewable Multi-Vitamins with Iron & Zinc	2.4	17	
National Vitamins	Dino-Life Chewable Multi-Vitamins with Extra C	2.4	17	
Plante International	Children's Choice Gummi Bear	2.3	16	
Kaire Essentials	Children's Chewables	2.2	16	
Vitamin Power	Children's Multi-Vites with Minerals	2.1	15	DOSAGE DERIVED

On A Personal Note

MacWilliam Communications is an independent Canadian company, specializing in health science research and publishing. Created in 1999, the company holds the copyright to its popular reference guide, the *Comparative Guide to Nutritional Supplements* (2003). The book is the sole creation of MacWilliam Communications Inc. and was not commissioned or funded by any nutritional manufacturer or other public or private agency. It is the culmination of intensive research by the author on nutritional products sold in the United States and Canada.

Mr. Lyle MacWilliam, CEO of MacWilliam Communications Inc., is an educator, author and biochemist who serves as a consultant, contributory writer and public advocate for the natural healthcare industry. His creative work is utilized by several leading nutritional manufacturers, including: Douglas Laboratories, Life Extension Foundation, Source Naturals, USANA Health Sciences and Vitamin Research Products. Mr. MacWilliam has also attended nutritional conferences as a speaker and sponsored guest of a number of these companies. A recognized public speaker, Mr. MacWilliam has presented seminars on nutritional health throughout Canada, the United States, Australia, New Zealand and Singapore.

As a consultant, Mr. MacWilliam's scientific, communications and research skills are available to, and have been solicited by, several nutritional companies and public agencies. A contributory writer for Life Extension Foundation, a non-profit organization dedicated to the scientific exploration of preventive health and longevity, he has also served as a consultant with: Health Canada; Environment Canada; Human Resources Development Canada; the British Columbia Science Council; and USANA Health Sciences. Mr. MacWilliam also recently served as a member of the Transition Team for the Office of Natural Health Products (Health Protection Branch), created to develop a new regulatory framework for natural health products sold in Canada.

MacWilliam Communications Inc. has no fiduciary ties to any of the products or manufacturers represented in its publications, nor does the company accept financial contributions from any agency in the production of its guides. Mr. MacWilliam does not sell or market any nutritional products, nor does he benefit in any direct or indirect manner from the sales or marketing of any nutritional supplements in Canada or elsewhere.